# Emergency Radiology Cases

D1614688

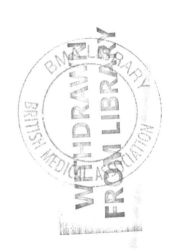

# Emergency Radiology Cases

Hani H. Abujudeh, MD, MBA, FSIR

Associate Professor of Radiology

Harvard Medical School

Massachusetts General Hospital

Boston, Massachusetts

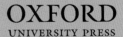

OXFORD

UNIVERSITY PRESS

# OXFORD
UNIVERSITY PRESS

Oxford University Press is a department of the University of Oxford.
It furthers the University's objective of excellence in research, scholarship,
and education by publishing worldwide.

Oxford   New York
Auckland   Cape Town   Dar es Salaam   Hong Kong   Karachi
Kuala Lumpur   Madrid   Melbourne   Mexico City   Nairobi
New Delhi   Shanghai   Taipei   Toronto

With offices in
Argentina   Austria   Brazil   Chile   Czech Republic   France   Greece
Guatemala   Hungary   Italy   Japan   Poland   Portugal   Singapore
South Korea   Switzerland   Thailand   Turkey   Ukraine   Vietnam

Oxford is a registered trademark of Oxford University Press
in the UK and certain other countries.

Published in the United States of America by
Oxford University Press
198 Madison Avenue, New York, NY 10016

Library of Congress Cataloging-in-Publication Data
Abujudeh, Hani H., author.
Emergency radiology cases / Hani Abujudeh.
    p. ; cm.—(Cases in radiology)
Includes bibliographical references and index.
ISBN 978–0–19–994117–9 (alk. paper)
I. Title.   II. Series: Cases in radiology.
[DNLM: 1. Diagnostic Imaging—Case Reports.   2. Emergency Medicine—Case
Reports.   3. Radiology—Case Reports. WN 180]
RC78.7.D53
616.07′54—dc23        2013022349

9 8 7 6 5 4 3 2 1
Printed in the United States of America
on acid-free paper

# Acknowledgments

The Publisher thanks the following for their time and advice:

Mark Anderson, University of Virginia
Sanjeev Bhalla, Mallinckrodt Institute of Radiology, Washington University
Michael Bruno, Penn State Hershey Medical Center
Melissa Rosado de Christenson, St. Luke's Hospital of Kansas City
Rihan Khan, University of Arizona
Angela Levy, Georgetown University
Alexander Mamourian, University of Pennsylvania
Stacy Smith, Brigham and Women's Hospital

# Preface

This book provides a concise, high-yield, imaging overview of the spectrum Emergency and Trauma conditions. The cases are presented in an easy-to-read format, including the most recent information. Although the book is not intended to be comprehensive it includes the most important presentations in the acute settings. The images are of high quality and include the most recent technologies, such as three-dimensional imaging. The book is divided into Trauma and Nontrauma Emergencies, and it is further subdivided by body regions. There is an additional section on Pediatric Emergency Cases. We hope this book will serve as a quick reference, and assist you in mastering Emergency Radiology.

Hani H. Abujudeh, MD, MBA, FSIR

# Contents

# Contributors

**Essmaeel Abdel-Dayem, MD**
South Shore Radiology Associates
Weymouth, Massachusetts
First Author: Cases 132, 136, 142, 146

**Hani H. Abujudeh, MD, MBA**
Associate Professor of Radiology
Harvard Medical School
Massachusetts General Hospital
Boston, Massachusetts
Book Editor: Emergency Radiology Cases
Senior Author: Cases 18, 21, 22, 24, 25 27,
    28, 30, 36, 38, 45, 46, 47, 49, 53, 54, 58, 59,
    60, 64, 66, 67, 69, 76, 78, 83, 95, 101, 111,
    115, 121, 124, 123, 125, 126, 127, 128, 129,
    130, 131, 132, 133, 134, 136, 137, 142, 146,
    149, 150, 151, 153, 155, 163, 164

**Tarik K. Alkasab, MD**
Instructor in Radiology
Department of Radiology
Massachusetts General Hospital
Boston, Massachusetts
Section Editor: Trauma - Abdomen
First Author: Cases 17, 20, 147, 148

**Shima Aran, MD**
Research Fellow
Department of Radiology
Massachusetts General Hospital
Boston, Massachusetts
First Author: Case 54

**Laura L. Avery, MD**
Assistant Professor of Radiology
Massachusetts General Hospital
Boston, Massachusetts
Part Editor: Nontrauma
First Author: Cases 13, 14, 15, 16

**Yolanda Bryce, MD**
Clinical Fellow in Radiology (EXT)
Department of Radiology
Mount Auburn Hospital
Cambridge, Massachusetts
First Author: Cases 25, 47, 76, 125, 127, 129,
    130, 133, 137, 153, 163, 164

**Judah G. Burns, MD**
Assistant Professor of Radiology
Division of Neuroradiology
Albert Einstein College of Medicine
Montefiore Medical Center
Bronx, New York
First Author: Cases 1, 2, 5

**Scott Cameron, MD**
Department of Diagnostic Imaging
Newport Hospital
Newport, Rhode Island
First author: Case 53, 149

**Carson Campe, MD**
Clinical Fellow in Radiology (EXT)
Department of Radiology
Massachusetts General Hospital
Boston, Massachusetts
Section Editor: Trauma - Upper Extremity
First Author: Cases 18, 22, 28, 58, 59, 60, 67
Senior Author: Cases 61, 65

**Enzo Cento, MD**
Advanced Radiology Services
Grand Rapids, Michigan
First Author: Cases 41, 44, 48, 96, 135, 138,
    154, 161

Robert Chen, MD
Instructor in Radiology
Department of Radiology
Massachusetts General Hospital
Boston, Massachusetts
First Author: Cases 68, 88, 97, 162

Garry Choy, MD
Instructor in Radiology
Department of Radiology
Massachusetts General Hospital
Boston, Massachusetts
Section Editor: Trauma - Chest
First Author: Cases 33, 34, 35, 37, 113, 114,
    118, 122, 123

Ryan M. Christie, MD
Assistant Professor of Radiology
Division of Emergency Radiology
Emory University School of Medicine
Atlanta, Georgia
First Author: Cases 29, 31, 32

Laleh Daftari Besheli
Research Fellow
Department of Radiology
Massachusetts General Hospital
Boston Massachusetts
First Author: Case 150

Dameon Duncan, MD
Assistant Professor of Radiology
Department of Radiology
Albert Einstein College of Medicine
Montefiore Medical Center
Bronx, New York
First Author: Case 116

R. Joshua Dym, MD
Assistant Professor of Radiology
Department of Radiology
Albert Einstein College of Medicine
Montefiore Medical Center
Bronx, New York
First Author: Cases 119, 120, 139, 141, 160

Daniel T. Ginat, MD
Instructor in Radiology
Department of Radiology
Massachusetts General Hospital
Boston, Massachusetts
First Author: 10, 100, 107, 108

Andrew J. Gunn, MD
Clinical Fellow in Radiology (EXT)
Department of Radiology
Massachusetts General Hospital
Boston, Massachusetts
First Author: Cases 30, 36, 95, 115, 121, 128,
    131, 134

Harlan B. Harvey, MD
Clinical Fellow in Radiology (EXT)
Department of Radiology
Massachusetts General Hospital
Boston, Massachusetts
First Author: Cases 21, 24, 49, 101, 151

Rania Hitto MD
Clinical Fellow
Division of Neuro-Radiology
Massachusetts General Hospital
Boston, Massachusetts
First Author: Case 112

Luke F. M. Hoagland, MD
Clinical Fellow in Radiology (EXT)
Department of Radiology
Massachusetts General Hospital
Boston, Massachusetts
First Author: Cases 46, 124, 155

Jamlik O. Johnson, MD
Assistant Professor of Radiology
Division Director for Emergency Radiology
Emory University School of Medicine
Atlanta, Georgia
Section Editor: Nontrauma - Abdomen
First Author: Cases 42, 43, 117, 140

Jason M. Johnson, MD
Instructor in Radiology
Department of Radiology
Massachusetts General Hospital
Boston, Massachusetts
Section Editor: Nontrauma - Head, Neck,
    and Spine
First Author: Cases 103, 104, 105, 106, 109, 110

Rathachai Kaewlai, MD
Department of Radiology
Bumrungrad International Hospital
Bangkok, Thailand
Part Editor: Trauma
First Author: Cases 92, 94

Christine Kassis, MD
Clinical Fellow in Radiology (EXT)
Department of Radiology
Massachusetts General Hospital
Boston, Massachusetts
First Author: Case 126

Taj Kattapuram, MD
Clinical Fellow in Radiology (EXT)
Department of Radiology
Massachusetts General Hospital
Boston, Massachusetts
First Author: Cases 27, 38, 66, 78, 111

Faisal Khosa, MD
Assistant Professor of Radiology
Division of Emergency Radiology
Emory University School of Medicine
Atlanta, Georgia
Senior Author: Cases 39, 40, 55, 145

Mykol Larvie
MDInstructor in Radiology
Department of Radiology
Massachusetts General Hospital
Boston, Massachusetts
Section Editor: Trauma - Brain
First Author: Cases 3, 4, 7, 8, 9, 11, 87, 90,
    99, 102

Peter MacMahon, MD
Department of Radiology
Mater Misericordiae University Hospital
Dublin, Ireland
Section Editor: Trauma - Spine
First Author: Cases 56, 61, 62, 63, 65, 77, 79,
    80, 81, 82, 86

Louis Marone, MD
Clinical Fellow in Radiology (EXT)
Department of Radiology
Massachusetts General Hospital
Boston, Massachusetts
Section Editor: Nontrauma - Chest
First Author: Cases 19, 26

Timothy Meehan, MD
Clinical Fellow in Radiology (EXT)
Department of Radiology
Massachusetts General Hospital
Boston, Massachusetts
First Author: Cases 45, 64, 69

Parul Penkar, MD
Instructor in Radiology
Department of Radiology
Massachusetts General Hospital
Boston, Massachusetts
First Author: Cases 70, 71, 72, 73, 74, 75,
    84, 85

Otto Rapalino, MD
Instructor in Radiology
Department of Radiology
Massachusetts General Hospital
Boston, Massachusetts
First Author: Cases 89, 91, 98

Marianne Reed, MD
Diagnostic Radiology
Yale-New Haven Hospital
New Haven, Connecticut
Senior Author: Cases 103, 105, 106, 109, 110

Javier M. Romero, MD
Assistant Professor of Radiology
Department of Radiology
Massachusetts General Hospital
Boston, Massachusetts
First Author: Cases 6, 12, 93

Pamela W. Schaefer, MD
Director, MR Imaging
Associate Director, Neuroradiology
Massachusetts General Hospital
Boston, Massachusetts
Section Editor: Nontrauma - Brain

Meir H. Scheinfeld, MD, PhD
Assistant Professor, Department of Radiology
Albert Einstein College of Medicine
Director, Division of Emergency Radiology
Montefiore Medical Center
Bronx, New York
First Author: Case 57

J. Gabriel Schneider, MD
Clinical Fellow in Radiology (EXT)
Department of Radiology
Massachusetts General Hospital
Boston, Massachusetts
Section Editor: Trauma–Lower Extremity
First Author: Case 50

**Randheer Shailam, MD**
Instructor in Radiology
Department of Radiology
Massachusetts General Hospital
Boston, Massachusetts
Part Editor: Pediatric
First Author: Cases 152, 156, 157, 158, 159

**Michael Spektor**
Assistant Professor in Radiology
Department of Radiology
Albert Einstein College of Medicine
Montefiore Medical Center
Bronx, New York
First Author: Case 144

**Freddie Swain, MD**
Assistant Professor of Radiology
Division of Emergency Radiology
Emory University School of Medicine
Atlanta, Georgia
First Author: Cases 39, 40, 55, 145

**Adam Ulano, MD**
Resident in Radiology
Mount Auburn Hospital
Cambridge, Massachusetts
First Author: Case 83

**Jason Weiden, MD**
Assistant Professor of Radiology
Division of Emergency Radiology
Emory University School of Medicine
Atlanta, Georgia
First Author: Cases 23, 51, 52, 143

# Part I    Trauma

# Section 1  Head and Face

**History**

▶ None

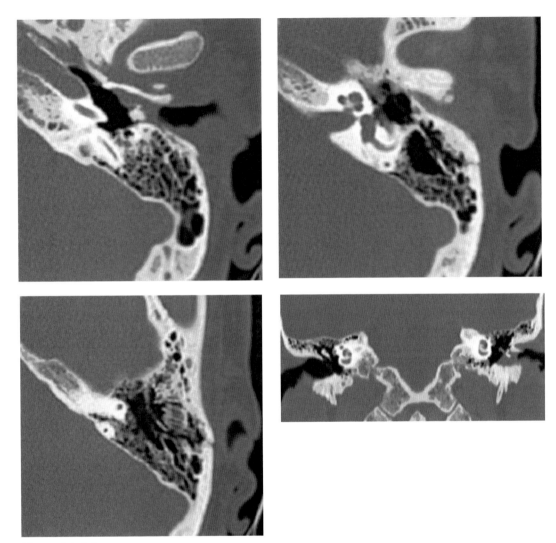

**Figures 1.1–1.4**

# Case 1  Temporal Bone Fracture (Longitudinal)

## Findings

▸ Imaging checklists
- Fractures classified into three types: longitudinal, transverse, and mixed/oblique
- Middle ear ossicles (most common ossicular injuries involve the incus and its articulations)
- Otic capsule (involvement increases risk of SNHL, facial nerve injury, CSF leak)
- Carotid canal (involvement should prompt evaluation for ICA dissection or occlusion)

▸ On MRI, T1W hyperintensity can be used to assess for middle ear or labyrinthine hemorrhage

## Differential Diagnosis

▸ Pseudofracture: Multiple sutures, fissures, and aqueducts course through the temporal bone
- Typically bilateral, symmetric, and corticated margins

## Teaching Points

▸ Fracture through temporal bone, often with associated facial nerve injury or ossicular involvement
▸ Three types of fractures
- Longitudinal: Parallels long axis of petrous bone; higher risk of ossicular dislocation
- Transverse: Perpendicular to long axis of petrous bone; higher risk of facial nerve injury
- Mixed/oblique type

▸ Communication between middle ear and membranous labyrinth caused by oval/round window rupture is called perilymphatic fistula

## Management

▸ Conservative management is usual first-line therapy. Many CSF leaks spontaneously resolve. Carefully monitor for possible meningitis.

### Further Readings

Dahiya R, Keller JD, Litofsky NS, Bankey PE, Bonassar LJ, Megerian CA. Temporal bone fractures: otic capsule sparing versus otic capsule violating clinical and radiographic considerations. *J Trauma.* 1999;47(6):1079–1083.

Saraiya PV, Aygun N. Temporal bone fractures. *Emerg Radiol.* 2009;16(4):255–265.

**History**

▶ Fall at nursing home.

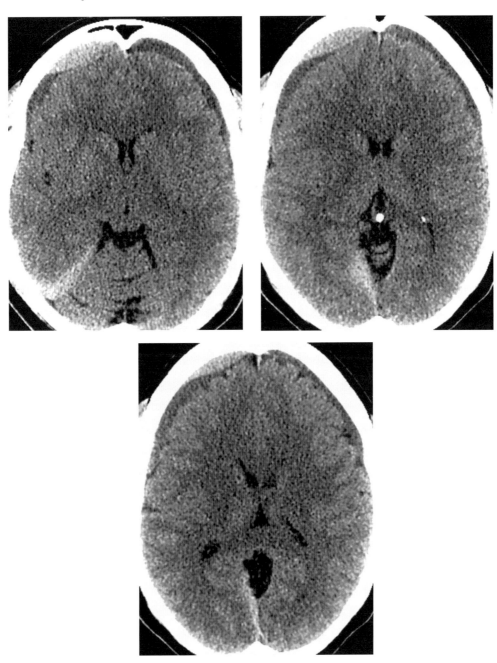

**Figures 2.1–2.3**

# Case 2  Acute Subdural Hematoma

### Findings

#### CT

- ▶ Crescentic, hyperdense collection within the extra-axial space that can cross suture lines but limited by dural attachments
- ▶ Pitfalls on CT
  - ▪ Acute SDH may be heterogeneous or low in density
  - ▪ Mixed-density subdural can be seen with clot retraction or arachnoid tear
  - ▪ Isodense subdural may be present with anemia or subacute hemorrhage

#### MRI

- ▶ Variable signal intensity on T1W/T2W imaging; hyperintense on FLAIR
- ▶ Displaced bridging veins often visible with contrast

### Differential Diagnosis

- ▶ Epidural hematoma: Lenticular (biconvex) extra-axial hemorrhage, limited by suture lines (may cross dural attachments); associated skull fracture often seen on CT
- ▶ Hygroma: simple CSF collection in subdural space
- ▶ Empyema: Peripherally enhancing, infected collection of pus; restricted diffusion on DWI

### Teaching Points

- ▶ Acute collection of blood products between the inner layer of the dura and arachnoid membranes
- ▶ Acute hemorrhage is usually as a result of severe head trauma, high-velocity acceleration, or deceleration head injury. Chronic SHD is usually caused by more trivial trauma in patients with risk factors (chronic alcoholism, epilepsy, coagulopathy).
- ▶ In children, neonatal hematomas may be related to delivery, and usually resolve. In infants and toddlers, nonaccidental trauma must be considered.
- ▶ Typically overlies convexity, although posterior fossa hemorrhages can occur
- ▶ SDHs may be symptomatic even when small, especially in young patients
- ▶ Density characteristics are not an absolute indicator of relative timing of hemorrhage

### Management

- ▶ Careful neurologic monitoring with expectant surgical management

### Further Readings

Freeman WD, Aguilar MI. Intracranial hemorrhage: diagnosis and management. *Neurol Clin.* 2012;30(1):211–240.
Barnes PD. Imaging of nonaccidental injury and the mimics: issues and controversies in the era of evidence-based medicine. *Radiol Clin North Am.* 2011;49(1):205–229.

**History**

▶ 46-year-old male who fell down stairs.

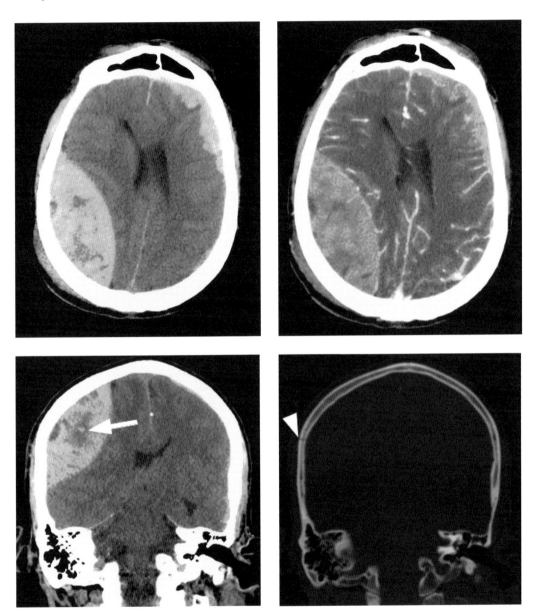

**Figures 3.1–3.4**

# Case 3  Epidural Hematoma

## Findings
### CT

▶ A large right parietal epidural hematoma involving rupture of the right middle meningeal artery causes severe mass effect, including leftward midline shift

▶ Heterogeneous density within the hematoma reflects recent and possibly active extravasation (arrow)

▶ There is a nondisplaced fracture in the right parietal bone (arrowhead)

▶ The anteroinferior margin of the right parietal epidural hematoma is bounded by the right temporoparietal suture

▶ There is a smaller left frontotemporal subdural hematoma

### CTA (lower right image)

▶ Dural and superficial cortical vessels are displaced away from the calvarium by the epidural hematoma

## Clinical Presentation

▶ Most commonly associated with major head trauma

▶ Epidural hematomas may develop over time, resulting in a lucid interval during which the patient is less symptomatic followed by more profound impairment

## Pathophysiology

▶ Intracranially, the dura is the periosteum and epidural hemorrhage requires the dissection of the dura away from its calvarial attachment

▶ Epidural hematomas are most commonly related to arterial rupture and are frequently seen in the setting of calvarial fractures, with increased frequency related to displaced fractures

▶ Epidural hematomas may also arise from venous disruption

▶ Middle meningeal artery branches in the temporal and parietal regions are vulnerable to injury, and most epidural hematomas occur in these regions

## Teaching Points

▶ Major head trauma, calvarial fracture, and a lucent interval followed by more profound impairment are features concerning for epidural hematoma

▶ Epidural hematoma does not typically cross sutures unless there is severe fracture at the suture line

▶ Large epidural hematomas are typically lentiform in configuration, although small epidural hematomas may conform to local boundaries

▶ Postcontrast images may show active extravasation

## Management

▶ Patients with even small epidural hematomas must be carefully monitored, because progressive bleeding may rapidly become life threatening

▶ Medical therapy should be directed toward maintaining cerebral perfusion pressure, and may include volume resuscitation, osmotic diuretics, and hyperventilation

▶ Surgical drainage may be achieved with burr holes or craniectomy

**History**

► 72-year-old female in motor vehicle collision with closed head trauma.

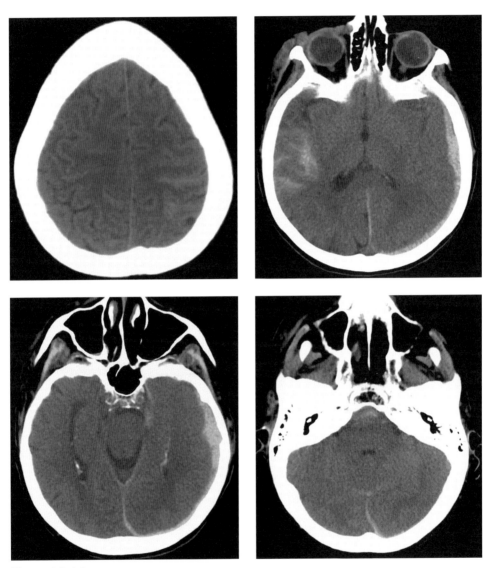

**Figures 4.1–4.4**

# Case 4  Subarachnoid Hemorrhage

## Findings

▶ Hyperdensity consistent with subarachnoid hemorrhage (SAH) outlining the left precentral gyrus (upper left)
▶ SAH outlining the right sylvian fissure and infiltrating sulci in the right temporal lobe (upper right)
▶ Trace intraventricular hemorrhage layering in the occipital horn of the right lateral ventricle (lower left)
▶ SAH in the prepontine cistern (lower right)
▶ Subdural hematoma overlying the left temporal, parietal, and occipital lobes and extending along the falx and left tentorial leaflet (multiple images)

## Clinical Presentation

▶ Common symptoms include headache, nausea and vomiting, and decreased consciousness

## Pathophysiology

▶ The arachnoid mater overlies the pia mater, which is the deepest layer of the meninges covering the brain and spinal cord, and SAH expands the space between these coverings
▶ The pia mater is extensively innervated with nerve fibers that transmit pain and are irritated by blood, resulting in severe headache, such as a thunderclap headache
▶ Intraventricular hemorrhage is a subtype of SAH

## Teaching Points

▶ Head CT is the most appropriate first examination to evaluate for SAH
▶ Lumbar puncture is often more sensitive than CT for SAH, and may reveal evidence of chronic SAH, such as xanthochromia
▶ MRI is relatively less sensitive for early SAH, although very sensitive for chronic SAH, which produces a strong susceptibility signal
▶ Traumatic SAH is strongly associated with other forms of traumatic brain injury, including contusion and diffuse axonal image

## Management

▶ The diagnosis of traumatic SAH requires exclusion of nontraumatic SAH, which may precipitate subsequent trauma (e.g., a fall or motor vehicle collision)
▶ When there is any consideration that nontraumatic SAH is present, vascular imaging with CT angiography is indicated to evaluate for intracranial aneurysm, the leading cause of nontraumatic SAH
  ▪ Complications of SAH that warrant close observation
  ▪ SAH may impair CSF resorption and lead to increased intracranial pressure and hydrocephalus
  ▪ SAH can cause vasospasm, typically within 4–10 days, that may result in territorial ischemia
  ▪ Hunt & Hess classification grades the clinical presentation from 1 (mildest) to 5 (most severe)
  ▪ Fischer grade classifies the quantity and location of SAH on CT from 1 (none evident) to 4 (diffuse or intraventricular or intraparenchymal extension)

## History

▶ Motor vehicle accident.

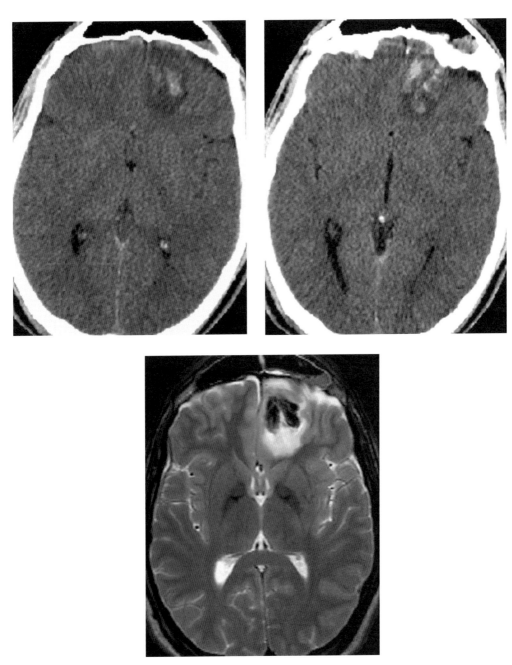

**Figures 5.1–5.3**

# Case 5  Cerebral Contusion

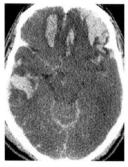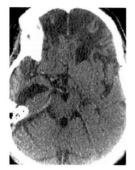

**Figures 5.4–5.5**

## Findings

### CT

▶ Cortical hyperattenuation
▶ Subcortical white matter swelling that is progressive over time

### MRI

▶ Cortical swelling
▶ Variable signal intensity of patchy hemorrhages, "blooming" on GRE sequences
▶ Bilateral, asymmetric injury is common
▶ May be accompanied by other forms of intracranial injury: subdural/epidural hematoma, fracture, contrecoup injury
▶ May result in chronic encephalomalacia

## Differential Diagnosis

▶ Cerebral infarction
▶ Infiltrative tumor (usually low grade); distinguished by clinical history
▶ Early cerebritis

## Teaching Points

▶ Posttraumatic brain injury with cortical and white matter injury often associated with coup-contrecoup injury and may be found distant from the site of impact
▶ Edema and patchy hemorrhage are common
▶ Hemorrhagic progression of contusion after initial trauma can result in severe, long-term loss of function in affected brain areas
▶ Characteristic locations adjacent to irregular skull surfaces
  ▪ Anterior, inferior frontal lobes
  ▪ Anterior temporal lobes
  ▪ Parasagittal (interhemispheric falx)
▶ The characteristic location of cerebral contusion can often differentiate this lesion from other infectious or neoplastic etiologies

## Management

▶ Supportive ICU care is paramount, with efforts aimed to optimize cerebral perfusion pressure and prevent seizures
▶ Strategies include administration of mannitol, hyperventilation, and sedation
▶ The use of antiepileptic medications may prevent early onset seizures, which can cause irreversible status epilepticus or increase intracranial pressure; however, may not prevent the later onset of epilepsy

## Further Readings

Alahmadi H, Vachhrajani S, Cusimano MD. The natural history of brain contusion: an analysis of radiological and clinical progression. *J Neurosurg.* 2010;112(5):1139–1145.

Kurland D, Hong C, Aarabi B, Gerzanich V, Simard JM. Hemorrhagic progression of a contusion after traumatic brain injury: a review. *J Neurotrauma.* 2012;29(1):19–31.

**History**

► None

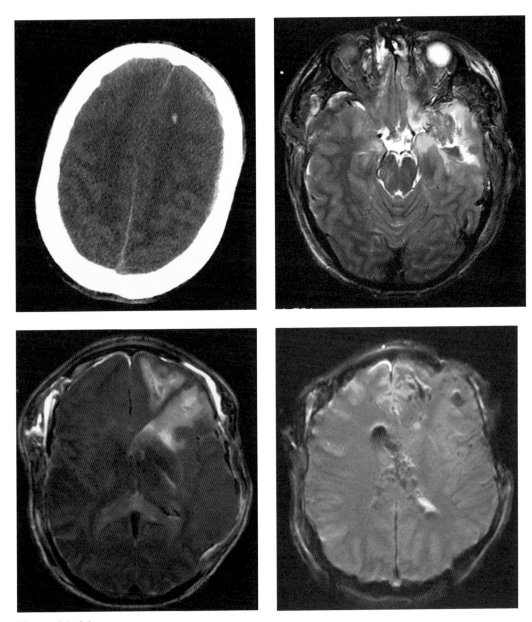

**Figures 6.1–6.4**

# Case 6  Diffuse Axonal Injury

### Findings

### CT

▶ Multiple hyperattenuated foci measuring 1–15 mm, typically in the cortical-subcortical junction, corpus callosum, and brainstem.

▶ These lesions may present a hypodense halo that likely represents peripheral edema.

▶ Sulci effacement may be present, with blurring of the gray and white matter interphase representing brain edema.

### MRI

▶ Multiple foci of blooming in GRE and SW images.

▶ Restricted diffusion in the cortical-subcortical junction, corpus callosum and brainstem.

▶ High T2/FLAIR signal in the areas of injury.

▶ The splenium is the segment most frequently involved of the corpus callosum.

▶ Brainstem involvement has a very poor clinical prognosis.

### Teaching Points

▶ Patients usually lose conscience and likely persist with altered mental status when they suffer DAI.

▶ This lesion is the result of traumatic acceleration/deceleration or rotational injuries.

▶ The degree of DAI severity is associated with the location of the injury. In ascending order of severity: cortical subcortical junction, corpus callosum, and brainstem.

▶ Brainstem DAI results in high mortality.

▶ Facial or skull fractures are not always associated with this type of trauma.

### Management

▶ Supportive ICU care is paramount, with efforts aimed to optimize cerebral perfusion pressure and prevent seizures.

▶ Strategies including administration of mannitol, hyperventilation, and sedation are important for the control of brain edema.

▶ The use of antiepileptic medications may prevent early onset seizures.

## History

▸ 52-year-old male with thrombocytopenia who fell from a bar stool.

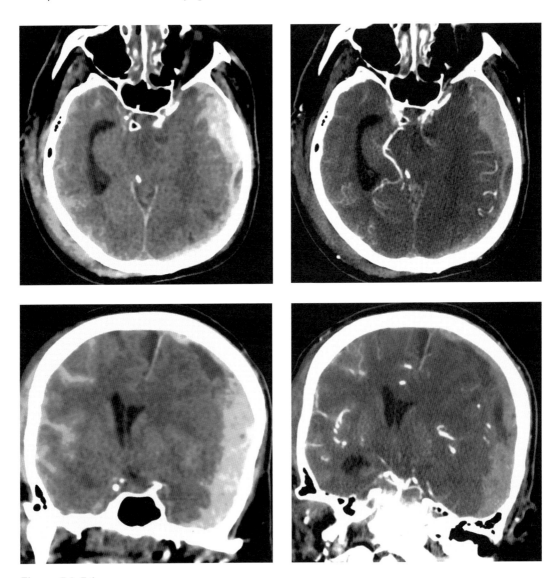

**Figures 7.1–7.4**

# Case 7  Intracranial Herniation

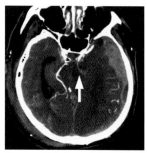 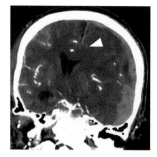

**Figures 7.5–7.6**

## Findings

### CT

▸ A large left cerebral subdural hematoma causes severe mass effect and brain herniation.

▸ The medial aspect of the left temporal lobe (the uncus) is displaced rightward across the tentorium, resulting in left uncal herniation.

▸ Portions of the left cerebral hemisphere, principally the left cingulate gyrus and the corpus callosum, are displaced to the right beneath the falx cerebri, resulting in subfalcine (or cingulate) herniation.

### CTA

▸ Left uncal herniation results in compression of the posterior cerebral artery (PCA) and posterior communicating artery (axial image, arrow). This may result in PCA territory infarction.

▸ Subfalcine herniation results in compression of the anterior cerebral arteries (ACAs). Normal right ACAs are present, whereas the left the ACAs are highly attenuated (coronal image, arrowhead). This may result in ACA territory infarction.

▸ Additional types of brain herniation (not depicted) include
  ▪ Upward or downward transtentorial herniation of the thalami, brainstem, and medial temporal lobes (central herniation)
  ▪ Cerebellar tonsil herniation through the foramen magnum
  ▪ Transcalvarial herniation, in which a portion of the brain protrudes through a defect in the calvarium that may be congenital, traumatic, or postsurgical

## Teaching Points

▸ Acute brain herniation requires emergent treatment

▸ May be caused by
  ▪ Intrinsic processes: intra-axial hemorrhage, edema or tumor
  ▪ Extrinsic processes: extra-axial hemorrhage, tumor, trauma
  ▪ Hydrocephalus or ventricular entrapment
  ▪ Compression of cerebral arteries may cause infarction
  ▪ Subfalcine herniation: ACA territory infarction
  ▪ Uncal herniation: PCA territory infarction
  ▪ Uncal herniation may impinge cranial nerves, particularly the third cranial nerves

## Management

▸ Intracranial pressure monitoring is indicated when there are signs, symptoms, or circumstances concerning for elevated intracranial pressure

▸ Medical: hypertonic saline, mannitol

▸ Surgical: hemicraniectomy

## Further Readings

Andrews BT. The recognition and management of cerebral herniation syndromes. In: Loftus CM, ed. *Neurosurgical Emergencies*. 2nd ed. New York: Thieme; 2008:34–44.

Ropper AH. Hyperosmolar therapy for raised intracranial pressure. *N Engl J Med*. 2012;367:746–752.

## History

▸ 51-year-old found down with ethanol intoxication.

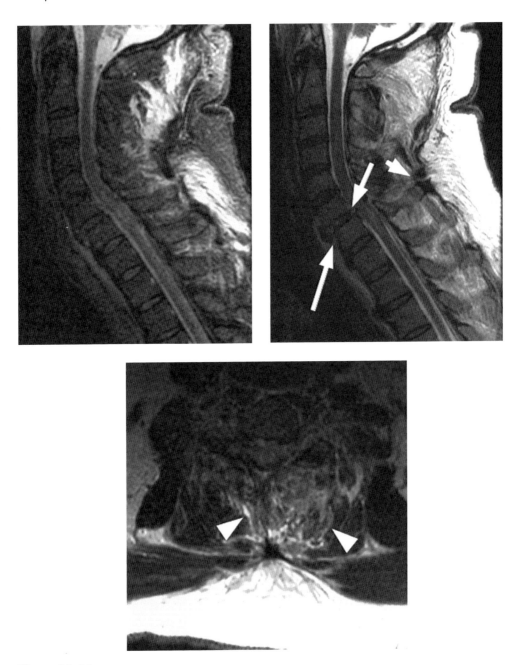

**Figures 8.1–8.3**

# Case 8   Spine Ligamentous Injury

## Findings

- Subtle anterolisthesis of the C5 and C6 vertebrae
- Disruption of the anterior longitudinal ligament, posterior longitudinal ligament, and supraspinous ligament (Figure 8.2; long, medium, and short arrows, respectively)
- Prevertebral soft tissue swelling from C6 through T3
- Extensive T2 hyperintensity consistent with edema in the posterior paraspinal muscles (Figure 8.3; arrowheads)
- Extensive edema in the posterior paraspinal soft tissues extending from the occiput superiorly through T2 inferiorly (Figure 8.1)
- T2 hyperintensity consistent with edema in the spinal cord at C6 through C7 reflecting spinal cord injury (see Case 9)
- Signal hyperintensity between spinous processes from C4 through T1 indicates injury to the interspinous ligamentous

## Clinical Presentation

- Spine ligamentous injury may occur with relatively mild trauma, such as fall from standing height and low-speed motor vehicle collisions
- Point tenderness may relate to spine ligamentous injury, although this is not a sensitive or specific finding for such

## Spectrum of Imaging Findings

- Alignment abnormality
  - Anterior, posterior, and lateral spondylolisthesis
  - Widening of spinous processes
- Intervertebral disk disruption
- Frank disruption of ligaments
- Edema in paraspinal soft tissues
- Epidural hematoma, particularly in relation to disruption of the posterior longitudinal ligament
- Craniocervical junction injuries
  - Apical ligament
  - Alar ligaments
  - Cruciate ligaments
  - Tectorial membrane
  - Anterior and posterior atlantooccipital membranes
  - Posterior atlantoaxial membrane

## Teaching Points

- Spine ligamentous injury is more apparent when imaged early, such as within 72 hours of injury, before edema begins to resolve
- In the cervical (C3-C7), thoracic and lumbar spine, two of three columns intact (anterior, posterior, and middle) is generally regarded as mechanically stable

## Management

- Immobilization of the entire spinal column is essential until spine is cleared
- Immobilization with braces is the mainstay of therapy for spine ligamentous injury without accompanying bone or spinal cord injury
- Nonsteroidal anti-inflammatory drugs are useful for pain control
- Surgery reserved to restore mechanical instability

## History

▶ 36-year-old male who fell two stories.

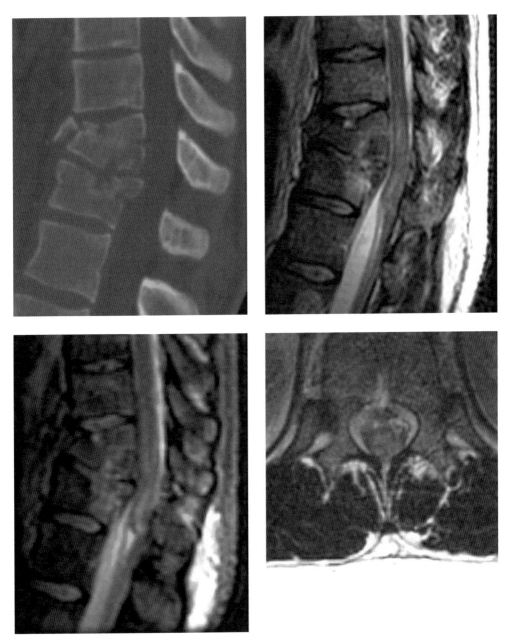

**Figures 9.1–9.4**

# Case 9  Spinal Cord Injury

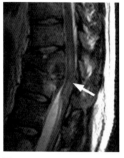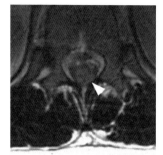

**Figures 9.5–9.6**

## Findings

### CT

▶ Comminuted fractures of the T11 and T12 vertebral bodies resulting in retropulsion of bone fragments into the spinal canal and loss of vertebral body height

### MRI

▶ Vertebral body fractures with bone marrow edema
▶ Abnormal expansion and edema in the inferior spinal cord consistent with acute contusion, prominently involving the conus medullaris (Figure 9.5; arrow)
▶ Edema in the central spinal cord and posterior columns (Figure 9.6; arrowhead)

## Clinical Presentation

▶ Symptoms are proportional to the severity of injury and level of spinal cord involvement
▶ High cervical SCI may cause coma and death because of brainstem injury
▶ Spinal cord injury without radiographic abnormality (SCIWORA): SCI occurring in the absence of abnormality detectable on plain radiographs or CT imaging
▶ SCIWORA most commonly occurs in children and frequently results in delayed presentation of even severe symptoms, such as paralysis

## Pathophysiology

▶ Acute SCI most commonly arises from trauma and involves intramedullary edema and often hemorrhage
▶ Nonacute SCI may arise from chronic trauma, most frequently in the setting of degenerative disk changes, resulting in spondylomyelopathy

## Teaching Points

▶ The degree of SCI may be disproportionate to spinal canal narrowing, because cord injury may result from transient deformations, as with SCIWORA
▶ Both acute and nonacute SCI may be present, especially in patients with significant degenerative changes
▶ Spinal cord edema may increase substantially in SCI, whereas hemorrhage generally does not

## Management

▶ Immobilization of the entire spinal column is essential until spine is cleared
▶ Prompt glucocorticoid administration reduces injury
▶ Loss of motor function is an indication for urgent surgical decompression
▶ Spine MRI is indicated in patients with neurologic deficits and for evaluation of obtunded patients

### Further Readings

Chandra J, Sheerin F, Lopez de Heredia L, Meagher T, King D, Belci M, Hughes RJ. MRI in acute and subacute post-traumatic spinal cord injury: pictorial review. *Spinal Cord.* 2012;50:2–7.

Chittiboina P, Cuellar-Saenz H, Notarianni C, Cardenas R, Guthikonda B. Head and spinal cord injury: diagnosis and management. *Neurol Clin.* 2012;30:241–276–ix.

**History**

▶ None

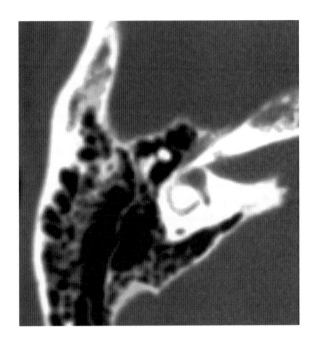

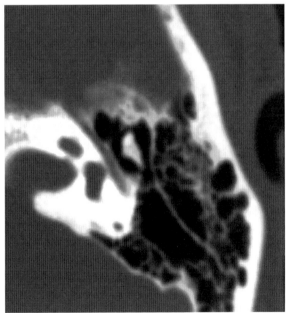

**Figures 10.1–10.2**

# Case 10   Ossicular Dislocation

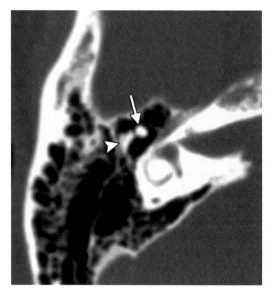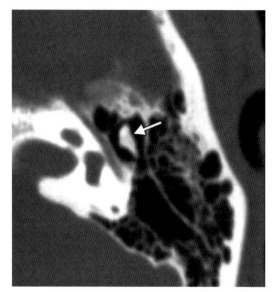

**Figures 10.3–10.4**

## Findings

▶ Figure 10.3 is an axial CT image of the right temporal bone that shows that the head of the malleus (arrow) is completely dissociated from the body of the incus (arrowhead).

▶ Figure 10.4 is an axial CT image of the corresponding normal left temporal bone that shows the intact ice-cream cone configuration of the incudomalleal joint (arrow).

## Differential Diagnosis

▶ Malleoincudal subluxation

▶ Incus interposition surgery

## Teaching Points

▶ Ossicular injury can lead to conductive hearing loss.

▶ The main types of ossicular disruption include incudomalleolar joint separation, incudostapedial joint separation, dislocation of the incus, dislocation of the malleoincudal complex, and stapediovestibular dislocation.

▶ Incudostapedial joint separation is the most common posttraumatic ossicular derangement, followed by complete incus dislocation from both its incudomalleolar and incudostapedial articulations.

▶ The incudomalleolar joint normally has an ice-cream cone configuration on axial CT images, in which the head of the malleus is seated in a groove (facet for the malleus) within the body of the incus. This arrangement is disrupted with incudomalleolar joint subluxation or dislocation and is therefore best appreciated on axial CT sections.

## Management

▶ Careful search for associated injuries on temporal bone CT, including temporal bone and ossicular fractures, perilymphatic fistula, and facial nerve injury.

▶ Ossiculoplasty.

## Further Readings

Meriot P, Veillon F, Garcia JF, Nonent M, Jezequel J, Bourjat P, Bellet M. CT appearances of ossicular injuries. *RadioGraphics*. 1997;17(6):1445–1454.

Yetiser S, Hidir Y, Birkent H, Satar B, Durmaz A. Traumatic ossicular dislocations: etiology and management. *Am J Otolaryngol*. 2008;29(1):31–36.

Zayas JO, Feliciano YZ, Hadley CR, Gomez AA, Vidal JA. Temporal bone trauma and the role of multidetector CT in the emergency department. *RadioGraphics*. 2011;31(6):1741–1755.

## History

► 86-year-old female who fell and injured her left face.

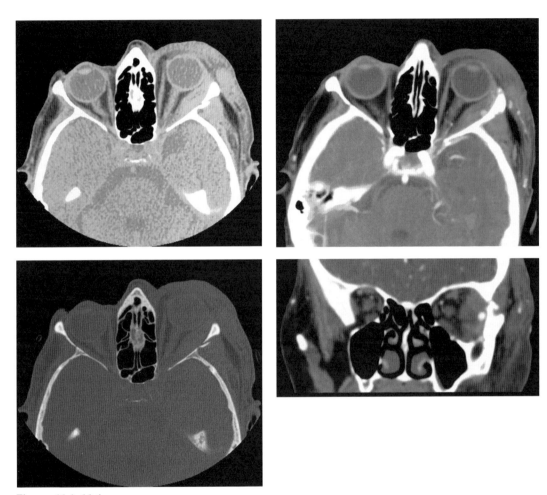

**Figures 11.1–11.4**

# Case 11  Orbital Hematoma

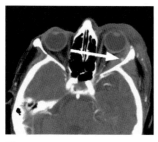 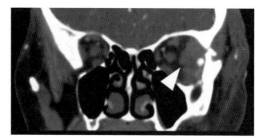

**Figures 11.5–11.6**

## Findings

### CT

- ► Preseptal, intraorbital density representing hematoma extending along the lateral orbital wall, with a convex margin projecting intraorbitally
- ► Mildly displaced fracture of the lateral orbital wall
- ► Marked mass effect contributing to mild proptosis
- ► Mild stretching of the optic nerve caused by proptosis
- ► Extensive preseptal periorbital soft tissue swelling

### CTA

- ► Punctate focus of contrast within the hematoma concerning for pseudoaneurysm or possibly active extravasation (Figure 11.5)
- ► Intraorbital displacement of the lateral rectus muscle (Figure 11.6)

## Clinical Presentation

- ► Commonly associated with trauma, especially blunt injury
- ► Clinical signs may include proptosis and decreased range of motion of the ipsilateral globe
- ► Clinical symptoms may include pain, decreased visual acuity, and diplopia resulting from decreased range of motion
- ► An afferent pupillary defect reflects nerve injury
- ► Surgical procedures that may cause orbital hematoma include endoscopic sinus surgery, blepharoplasty, and orbital reconstruction

## Pathophysiology

- ► In trauma, hemorrhage is most frequently subperiosteal related to disruption of small vessels in the periosteum
- ► Orbital hematomas may arise from extension of infection, particularly sinusitis, into the subperiosteal intraorbital space
- ► Less common causes of orbital hematoma include ruptured vascular malformation and hemorrhagic neoplasm
- ► Postseptal hemorrhage (posterior to the orbital septum) is more likely to cause injury to the globe, optic nerve, and other orbital structures than preseptal hematoma (anterior to the orbital septum)
- ► May cause an acute orbital compartment syndrome, which may lead to vision-threatening compressive optic neuropathy, which requires emergent management

## Teaching Points

- ► Traumatic and nontraumatic orbital hematomas most commonly occur in the subperiosteal space
- ► Active extravasation on postcontrast imaging is concerning for rapid expansion of the hematoma

## Management

- ► Conservative therapy may include glucocorticoids for anti-inflammatory effect, especially with delayed presentations
- ► Surgical treatment may involve hematoma evacuation and orbit reconstruction
- ► Hematoma evacuation may also be performed with needle aspiration

Further Reading

Ramakrishnan VR, Palmer JN. Prevention and management of orbital hematoma. *Otolaryngol Clin North Am.* 2010;43:789–800.

**History**

► None

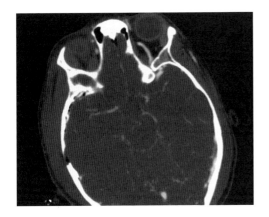 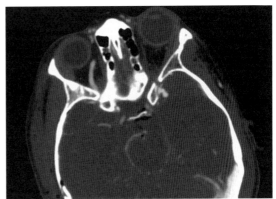

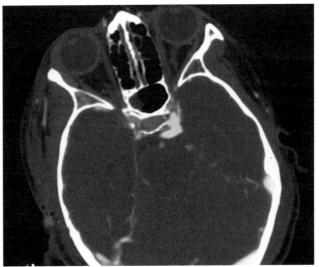

**Figures 12.1–12.3**

# Case 12  Carotid Cavernous Fistula

### CT

▶ There is bulging of the cavernous sinus
▶ Proptosis is noted ipsilateral to the fistula
▶ There is enlargement of the superior ophthalmic vein
▶ There is enlargement of the periorbital muscles

### CTA

▶ Enlargement and early contrast filling of the cavernous sinus
▶ Noticeable enlargement of the superior ophthalmic vein

### DSA

▶ Is the diagnostic gold standard
▶ Early filling of the petrosal sinus and ophthalmic vein is noted when the intracavernous carotid artery is injected
▶ Early contrast in the cavernous sinus

### Teaching points

▶ Patients may have tinnitus. At auscultation of the head, patients may have a bruit.
▶ The patient may experience diplopia and ophthalmoplegia (often from CN VI palsy).
▶ There could be visual loss caused by edema and blood shunting.
▶ CCF are divided in direct and indirect fistulas.

### Management

High-flow CCSF requires surgical repair or endovascular surgery. Current microcatheter techniques permit access to the cavernous sinus by several routes. Low-flow dural sinus CCSF that occurs spontaneously is very likely to resolve spontaneously.

   Surgical repair is considered in cases in which there is increased risk of vision loss (from glaucoma, corneal exposure, or posterior segment ischemia); new visual symptoms; or the development of headache.

**History**

▶ None

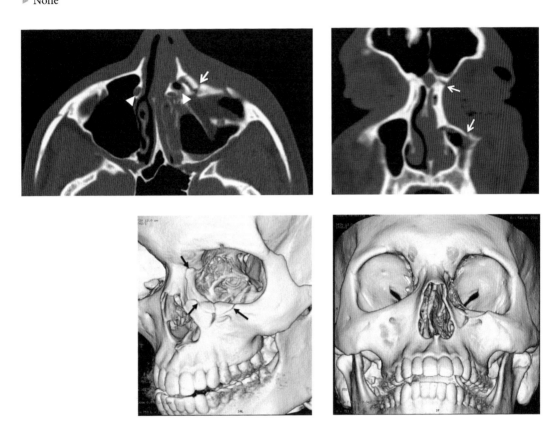

**Figures 13.1–13.4**

# Case 13  Left-sided Nasal Orbital Ethmoid Fracture

## Findings

▶ Figure 13.1. Axial image demonstrates comminuted fracture involving the inferior orbital rim with fracture through the base of the frontal process of maxilla (arrows). There is posterior displacement of the left nasolacrimal duct with extension of fracture to the duct with normal right-sided duct (arrowheads).

▶ Figure 13.2. Coronal image demonstrates a fracture through the nasal-frontal suture superiorly and fracture of the inferior orbital rim inferiorly. The orbital rim involvement is mildly comminuted.

▶ Figures 13.3, 13.4. Three-dimensional reformations give summary representation of nasal displacement and fracture of the orbital rim. Note well-demonstrated medial orbital fractures on the oblique image (black arrows).

## Differential diagnosis

▶ Nasal bone fractures.

## Teaching Points

▶ The naso-orbito-ethmoid (NOE) complex includes skeletal structures that are shared by both the nasal and orbital regions including the nasal bones, ethmoid bones and inferior orbital rims.

▶ Fractures commonly result in posterior displacement of the anterior nasal structures into the medial orbital rim and ethmoid sinuses, so-called telescoping.

▶ NOE fractures are clinically classified according to the degree of comminution of the central bone fragment of the orbital rim onto which the medial canthal tendon inserts. This tendon and related structures gives stability to the medial orbit and in cases of injury telecanthus can occur.

## Management

▶ Management of NOE fractures is typically with open reduction and internal fixation.

▶ The main goals are to restore the patient's appearance and to restore the anatomic position of the medial canthal tendon and the bony segment(s) to which it is attached.

▶ Attention may also be directed at repair or obliteration of the nasolacrimal duct if needed.

## Further Reading

Mehta N, Butala P, Bernstein MP. The imaging of maxillofacial trauma and its pertinence to surgical intervention. *Radiol Clin North Am.* 2012;50(1):43–57.

**History**

▶ None

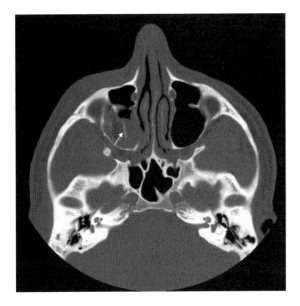
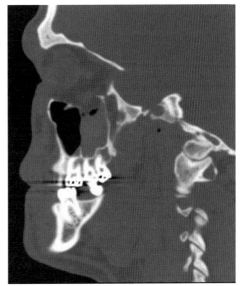
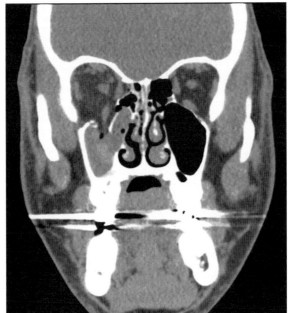

**Figures 14.1–14.3**

# Case 14  Right-Sided Orbital Floor Blow-Out Fracture

## Findings

► Axial image (Figure 14.1) at the level of the maxillary sinus shows opacification of the right maxillary sinus. A bone fragmentation of the orbital floor consistent with a fallen fragment (arrow) is identified with adjacent herniated intraorbital fat and layering blood.

► Sagittal image (Figure 14.2) demonstrates the large defect in the posterior orbital floor fracture with herniation of orbital contents.

► Coronal image (Figure 14.3) in soft tissue window demonstrates orbital floor fracture with "trapdoor" fragment medially and herniation of orbital fat into the defect. Inferior rectus is identified extending into the defect. Hyperintense blood products are identified in the maxillary sinus.

## Differential Diagnosis

None

## Teaching Points

► Orbital blow-out fractures result from direct blows to the orbit (fist, ball), which increase intraorbital pressure and result in fracture of the thin bony orbital lining (i.e., the floor or medial wall).

► The strong orbital rim remains intact with blow-out fractures.

► The fracture fragments and orbital soft tissue contents collapse outward into the air-filled sinus. When the extraocular muscles are involved and become herniated into the sinuses the globe may become entrapped. Significant increase in orbital volume and herniation of orbital fat may lead to enophthalmos and visual changes.

## Management

► Clinically significant indications for repair include entrapment and enophthalmos.

### Further Reading

Mehta N, Butala P, Bernstein MP. The imaging of maxillofacial trauma and its pertinence to surgical intervention. *Radiol Clin North Am*. 2012;50(1):43–57.

**History**

▸ None

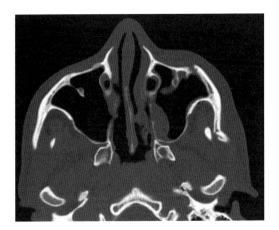
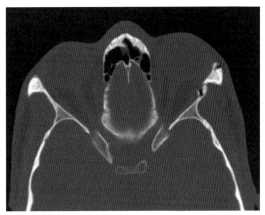
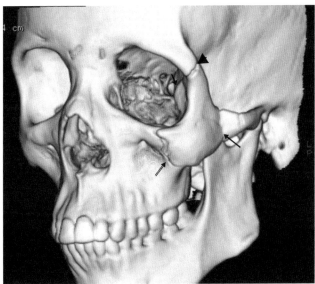

**Figures 15.1–15.3**

# Case 15 Zygoma Complex Fracture

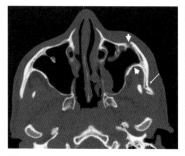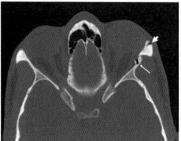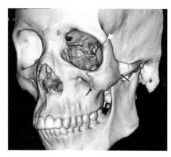

**Figures 15.4–15.6**

## Findings

▶ Axial image (Figure 15.4) demonstrates fracture of the anterior and posterior/lateral wall of the maxillary sinus at the zygomaticomaxillary sutures (arrowheads). Additionally, a fracture of the zygomatic arch with fracture of the zygomaticotemporal suture is seen (arrow).

▶ A superior axial image (Figure 15.5) through the level of the orbit demonstrates a fracture of the lateral orbital wall at the level of the zygomaticosphenoid suture (arrow). A more anterior fracture is seen as diastasis of the zygomaticofrontal suture (arrowhead). Frequently this fracture is best seen on coronal images.

▶ Slightly oblique three-dimensional image (Figure 15.6) demonstrates all four sutural attachments of the zygoma. The zygomaticotemporal suture (long arrow), the anterior zygomaticomaxillary suture (open arrow), the zygomaticofrontal suture (arrowhead), and the zygomaticosphenoid suture (short arrow).

## Differential Diagnosis

▶ Le Fort fractures

## Teaching Points

▶ A direct blow to the lateral midface (the zygomatic region) can result in disruption of the zygoma from its anatomic connections to the temporal, sphenoid, frontal, and maxillary bones.

▶ The zygomaticomaxillary involvement propagates through the infraorbital rim and orbital floor. This may result in globe entrapment.

▶ Depression of the zygomatic arch may result in compression of the underlying temporalis tendon at its insertion point on the coronoid process of the mandible, manifesting as trismus (limited mouth opening).

## Management

▶ The zygoma complex fracture may be reduced and fixated with malleable plates. Zygoma complex fractures are classified according to the direction and magnitude of displacement, and bony integrity of the zygoma, as originally described by Knight and North using plain films.

## Further Reading

Mehta N, Butala P, Bernstein MP. The imaging of maxillofacial trauma and its pertinence to surgical intervention. *Radiol Clin North Am.* 2012;50(1):43–57.

## History

▶ None

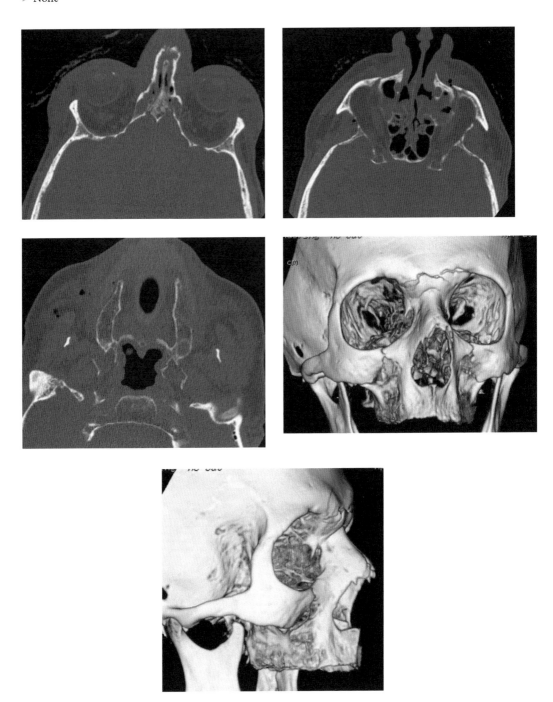

**Figures 16.1–16.5**

# Case 16   Le Fort Maxillary Fracture

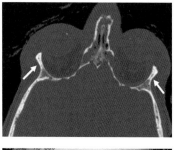
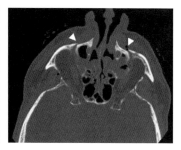
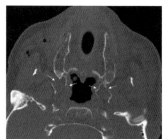
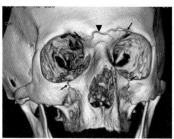
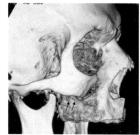

**Figures 16.6–16.10**

## Findings

### Le Fort II fracture

▶ Figure 16.6: Axial images of Le Fort II fracture demonstrates intact lateral orbital walls (arrows). The lateral orbital wall would be involved in a Le Fort III fracture.

▶ Figure 16.7: Inferior axial image demonstrates the orbital rims are fractured bilaterally (arrowheads), a finding in all Le Fort II fractures.

▶ Figure 16.8: Axial image more inferiorly demonstrates fractures of the pterygoid plates bilaterally (arrows).

▶ Figures 16.9 and 16.10: Three-dimensional images demonstrate fracture through the inferior and medial orbital rims (black arrows). A horizontal fracture is seen just superior to the nasofrontal suture (arrowhead). On sagittal view, note the propagation of the fracture through the posterior maxilla to involve the pterygoid plates (small black arrows).

## Differential Diagnosis

▶ Although naso-orbital-ethmoid fractures do include the inferior and medial orbital rims, they do not extend across the nasofrontal suture superiorly and do not involve the pterygoid plates.

▶ The Le Fort III fractures are a form of total cranial-facial disjunction and involve the zygoma and lateral orbital walls.

## Teaching Points

▶ All Le Fort maxillary fractures demonstrate fractures of the pterygoid plates.

▶ Le Fort I level extends horizontally at or just superior to the alveolar process of the maxilla with the fracture involving the anterior and posterior/lateral walls of the maxillary sinus. The nasal septum is also fractured. Clinically this fracture presents with a distinctly mobile palate relative to the remainder of the midface.

▶ Le Fort II fracture extends from the pterygoid plates to involve the inferior and medial orbital rims. Midline a fracture of the nasal bones or a diathesis at the nasofrontal suture occurs. The line of fracture includes the posterior/lateral and anterior walls of the maxillary sinus, the orbital floor, and the medial orbital wall. Clinically, the maxillary and nasal regions are mobile.

▶ Le Fort III, "craniofacial disjunction," the fracture line propagates from the pterygoid plates to involve the connection between the upper face and the skull base. Specifically, the fracture involves the pterygoid plates, zygomatic arches, lateral and medial orbital rims, and nasal bones or nasofrontal suture.

# Section 2 Spine

## History

▶ Motor vehicle accident.

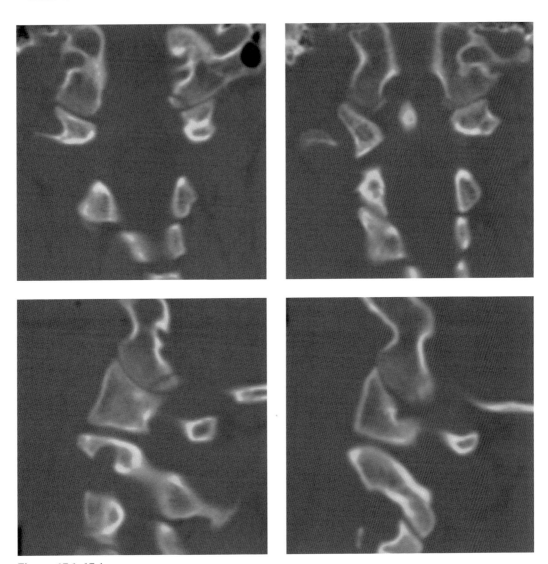

**Figures 17.1–17.4**

# Case 17   Occipital Condyle Fracture

## Findings

▶ Fracture lines extend through the occipital condyles as they touch the articular facets of C1, usually best seen in the coronal plane.
▶ Some fractures may be comminuted, with multiple small fragments.
▶ May see medial displacement of a smaller fracture fragment.
▶ May be associated with more complex skull base fractures or other cervical spine injuries.
▶ MRI may demonstrate disruption of craniocervical ligamentous structures.

## Differential Diagnosis

▶ Unfused apophyses/ossification centers
▶ Occipital condyle fracture

## Teaching Points

▶ Most frequently occurs in the context of other craniocervical injuries.
▶ Anderson and Montesano classification system
  ▪ Type I: Comminuted occipital condyle fracture, usually resulting from loading injury (similar to Jefferson fracture). Stable injury, with contralateral alar ligament intact.
  ▪ Type II: Extension of skull base fracture through the occipital condyle. Also considered stable, because ligamentous structures remain intact.
  ▪ Type III (most common): Avulsion fracture at the insertion of the alar ligament from the dens to the occipital condyle. Because of stress on the contralateral alar ligament, this is possibly an unstable injury.
▶ Tuli criteria for radiologic instability
  ▪ >8 degrees of occipitoatloid rotation
  ▪ >1 mm of occipitoatloid translation
  ▪ >7 mm of overhand of C2 on C1 (total both sides)
  ▪ >4-mm interval between anterior aspect of odontoid and posterior aspect of the anterior arch of C1
  ▪ <13-mm interval between posterior aspect of the odontoid and anterior aspect of the posterior arch of C1.
▶ CTA may be used to assess for vascular injury to the vertebral artery as it passes through the transverse groove of the atlas just posterior to the occipitoatloid articulations.
▶ MRI when a patient is stable is used to further assess the ligamentous structures, and assess for associated cord injury.
▶ Patients may experience nerve palsies of cranial nerves IX through XII because of involvement of these structures as they pass through the adjacent hypoglossal canal and jugular foramen.
▶ Management and clinical course is typically dictated by the associated injuries rather than the occipital condylar fractures as such.

## Management

▶ Typically dictated by associated injuries.
▶ Treatment options for unstable injuries may include surgical fixation or halo traction.

▸ None

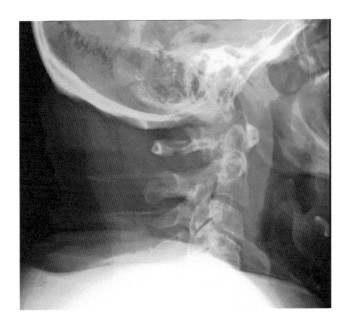

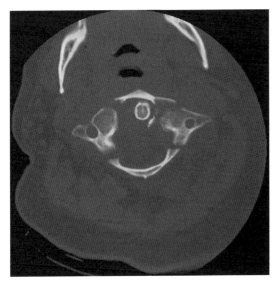

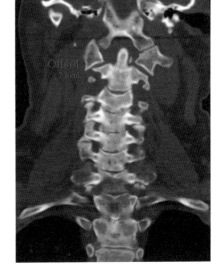

**Figures 18.1–18.3**

# Case 18   Jefferson Fracture

## Findings

▶ Burst fracture of the C1 vertebral body

### Radiograph

▶ Odontoid view: Offset between margins of C1 lateral masses and margins of subjacent C2 articular facets
  ▪ Combined offset >7 mm indicates rupture of transverse ligament
  ▪ May be normal variant in pediatric population
  ▪ Axial rotation can mimic offset
▶ Lateral view: Increased atlantodental interval on lateral
  ▪ Interval >6 mm indicates rupture of transverse ligament
▶ Flexion/Extension views
  ▪ Maybe required to evaluate integrity of transverse ligament and thus stability of fracture
▶ Beware of normal variants in pediatric population

### CT: Low threshold for CT

▶ Offset on odontoid view indication for CT
▶ Mechanism of trauma or symptoms is indication

## Differential Diagnosis

▶ Congenital variations in C1 arch fusion
▶ Pseudosubluxation of C1 on C2 without fracture

## Teaching Points

### Mechanism

▶ Axial loading: C1 vertebral body compressed between occipital condyles and C2 vertebral body resulting in forces that drive fracture fragments outward from central canal. Result is increased canal volume; spinal cord injury is rare.
▶ Hyperextension: Posterior arch fractures

### Fracture Subtypes

▶ Bilateral anterior or posterior arch fractures (single arch)
▶ Anterior and posterior arch fractures (includes classic Jefferson 4 part fracture)

## Lateral mass fracture

▶ Exclude congenital failure of fusion: three primary ossification sites that may not fuse

## Management

### Further Imaging

▶ CTA if suspicion of vertebral artery or PICA injury
  ▪ Extension of fracture into foramen transversarium
  ▪ Wallenberg syndrome (PICA)

### Transverse ligament integrity determines stability of fracture

▶ Transverse ligament disruption results in unstable fracture
▶ Imaging findings (above) determine suspicion for ligament rupture

### Treatment

▶ Stable fracture (intact transverse ligament): Cervical collar
▶ Unstable fracture (ruptured transverse ligament)
  ▪ Cervical traction and halo
  ▪ Surgery considered with increased displacement of C1/C2

## History

▶ 35-year-old female in high-velocity motor vehicle accident.

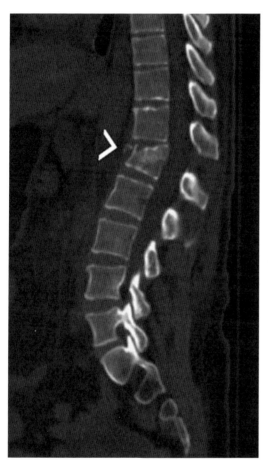 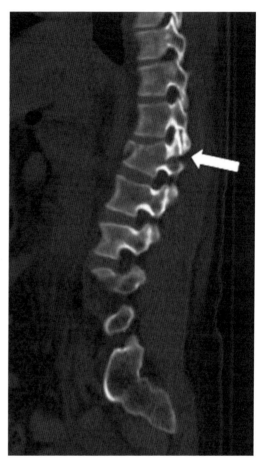

**Figures 19.1–19.2**

# Case 19   Chance Fracture

## Findings
### Radiograph
▶ Wedging of anterior vertebral body, focal kyphosis, widening of spinous processes.
▶ On AP radiograph, may see increased luceny of involved vertebral body, indicating a displaced spinous process (empty body sign).

### CT
▶ Vertebral body fracture with anterior wedging causing focal kyphosis (arrowhead).
▶ Transversely oriented fracture through posterior elements with increased interspinous distance (arrow).
▶ Uncovering of the articular facets (naked facet sign) secondary to distraction of the posterior elements.
▶ On axial images, may see gradual loss of pedicle definition (dissolving pedicle sign).
▶ May see retropulsion of fracture fragment into spinal canal, suggesting a burst component.

### MRI
▶ Hypointense fracture line on all sequences, with surrounding band of edema (sandwich sign).
▶ Disruption of interspinous and supraspinous ligaments.
▶ Spinal cord contusion, if present.

## Differential Diagnosis
▶ Shear injury
▶ Distraction injury
▶ Burst fracture
▶ Compression fracture
▶ Pathologic fracture

## Teaching Points
### Mechanism
▶ Flexion/distraction injury with compression of anterior column and distraction of middle and posterior columns, associated with use of the lap belt portion of a seat belt, which acts as a fulcrum around which the spine rotates during a motor vehicle accident.
▶ Most commonly occurs at T11-L3, but may occur in the midthoracic spine.
▶ Usually a mix of bony and soft tissue injury, with purely ligamentous Chance-type fractures rare.

### Associations
▶ Approximately 40% of patients with Chance-type fractures have associated intraabdominal injuries, of which bowel and mesentery injuries are most common.
▶ Focal neurologic deficits may or may not be present.
▶ Spinal cord injury especially if retropulsion of fragment into spinal canal.

### Management
▶ Often conservative with bracing despite initial instability of injury.
▶ Surgical fixation is indicated with increasing degrees of instability and ligamentous injury or if reduction cannot be maintained with bracing.

## History

▸ 67-year-old woman fell off horse, cannot turn head.

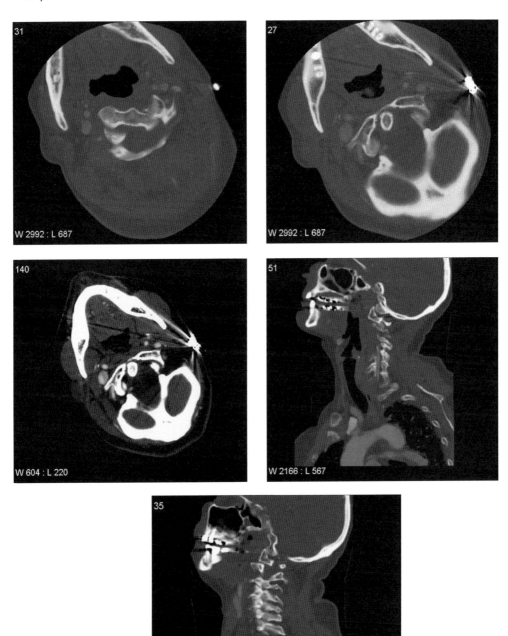

**Figures 20.1–20.5**

# Case 20  Atlantoaxial Rotatory Fixation

## Findings

- C1 is displaced with respect to C2, and rotated such that the C1 articular facet is anterior to the superior articular facet of C2.
- May also see fracture of the facets/articular processes associated with the impaction.
- Depending on relative displacement of C1 with respect to C2, may have marked narrowing of the canal.
- CTA may demonstrate cutoff or dissection of a vertebral artery.
- MRI may demonstrate associated ligamentous abnormality/disruption and elevated T2 signal in the cord.

## Differential Diagnosis

- Chronic atlantoaxial rotatory fixation
- Acute atlantoaxial rotatory fixation

## Teaching Points

- Hawkins and Fielding initially classified fixation by the degree of dissociation between the anterior arch of C1 and the odontoid
  - Type I: Normal distance between anterior arch and odontoid suggests lesser ligamentous injury.
  - Type II: 3–5 mm of anterior displacement of the anterior arch suggests transverse ligamentous injury.
  - Type III: >5 mm of anterior displacement suggests transverse and alar ligamentous injury.
  - Type IV: Posterior displacement of C1 with respect to C2.
- More recently, Pang has developed a classification system for chronic atlantoaxial rotatory fixation in pediatric patients that relies on a set of CT images of the atlantoaxial joint taken in at least three positions. This allows distinction between C1-C2 fixation and muscular torticollis.
- Acute, traumatic atlantoaxial rotatory fixation in adults is much rarer and clinically similar to facet dislocation/fracture at other levels.
- CTA should be considered to evaluate for a vascular injury of the vertebral arteries.

## Management

- Longitudinal traction and halo fixation can be used in acute cases.
- May require subsequent fusion of C1/C2 for stabilization.

### Further Readings

Rojas CA, Hayes A, Bertozzi JC, Guidi C, Martinez CR. Evaluation of the C1-C2 articulation on MDCT in healthy children and young adults. *AJR Am J Roentgenol*. 2009;193(5):1388–1392.

Booth TN. Cervical spine evaluation in pediatric trauma. *AJR Am J Roentgenol*. 2012;198(5):W417–W425.

Pang D. Atlantoaxial rotatory fixation. *Neurosurgery*. 2010;66(suppl 3):161–183.

## History

▶ None

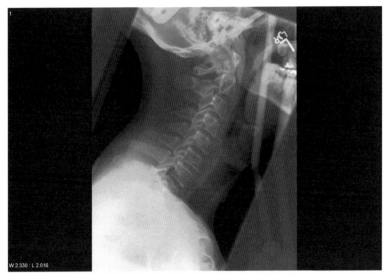

**Figures 21.1**

# Case 21 Hangman's Fracture

## Findings

### Radiography

▶ Anterior subluxation of C2 on C3
▶ Lucency through the posterior elements of C2 compatible with fracture
▶ Prevertebral soft tissue thickening

### CT

▶ Fractures of bilateral pars interarticulares of C2
▶ Involvement of the transverse foramen warrants CTA to rule out vertebral artery injury

## Differential Diagnosis

▶ Physiologic displacement of C2 on C3 in infants and young children
▶ Dens-arch synchondroses in children
▶ Primary spondylolyses in children

## Teaching Points

▶ Bilateral pars interarticularis fractures of C2 (axis)
▶ Hyperextension cervical spine injury
▶ Named hangman's fracture because during judicial hangings the executioner would place knot of the noose under the chin of the person being hung resulting in this injury pattern
  ▪ Nowadays, most injuries caused by face or chin hitting dashboard in a motor vehicle collision causing hyperextension and distraction
▶ Levine classification: (does not apply to children)
  ▪ Type I: <3 mm translation, no angulation
  ▪ Type II (most common): >3 mm translation, and >10 degrees of angulation
  ▪ Type III: all characteristics of type II + bilateral interfacetal dislocation
▶ Presentation
  ▪ Cervical spine point tenderness
  ▪ Absence of neurologic injury is common, because the fracture tends to expand the spinal canal preventing cord compression
  ▪ In very severe cases, the C3 body is subluxed posteriorly causing cord compression with devastating neurologic injury

## Management

▶ Halovest traction/immobilization for 12 weeks
▶ Surgical fusion for nonunion (rarely necessary)

Further Reading

Li XF, Dai LY, Lu H, Chen XD. A systematic review of the management of hangman's fractures. *Eur Spine J.* 2006;15(3):257–269.

**History**

► None

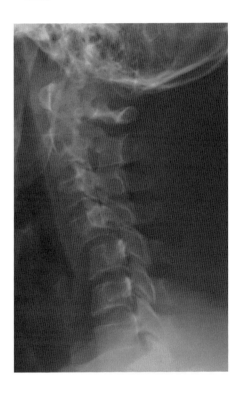
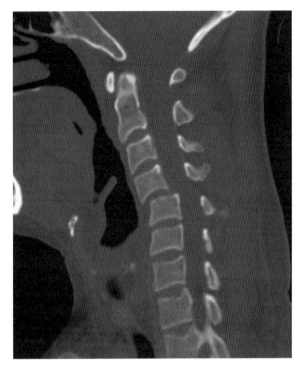

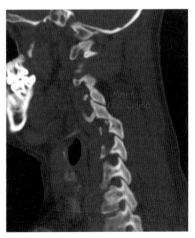
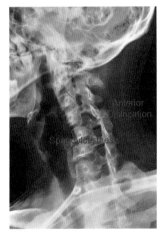
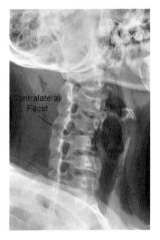

**Figures 22.1–22.5**

# Case 22  Unilateral Facet Dislocation of the Cervical spine

**Findings**

Anterior dislocation of inferior articular process relative to superior articular process of the caudal vertebral level

**Diagnosis**

- ▶ Radiographs: anteroposterior, lateral, and oblique
- ▶ CT with sagittal reconstructions
- ▶ Anterolisthesis of 25%–50%
    - ▪ If anterolisthesis >50% must suspect bilateral facet dislocation
- ▶ Assess patency of foramen transversarium
    - ▪ Risk of vertebral artery injury increased in hyperflexion injuries

**Associated Injuries**

- ▶ Fractures (ipsilateral or contralateral)
    - ▪ Lateral mass fracture
    - ▪ Articular process fractures
    - ▪ Transverse process fracture
    - ▪ Lamina fracture
- ▶ Contralateral facet injury
    - ▪ Fracture
    - ▪ Subluxation
- ▶ Posterior ligamentous injury (MRI)
    - ▪ Ligamentum flavum
    - ▪ Interspinous and superspinous ligaments
    - ▪ Posterior longitudinal ligament usually intact or at most partially torn, preventing further anterolisthesis
- ▶ Radiculopathy
    - ▪ Superior articular process rest in neural foramen after dislocation
- ▶ Cord injury RARE with unilateral facet dislocation
    - ▪ Stable injury when not accompanied by destabilizing fractures

**Differential Diagnosis**

- ▶ Bilateral facet dislocation
- ▶ Hyperflexion fracture

**Teaching Points**

**Mechanism**

- ▶ Hyperflexion-rotation
    - ▪ Most common in mid or lower cervical spine
- ▶ Axial rotation with fixed pivot point on one facet resulting in contralateral anterior dislocation

**Management**

- ▶ Closed reduction with cervical traction if neurologically intact
- ▶ Prereduction MRI if abnormal neurologic examination or altered mental state
- ▶ Surgery if
    - ▪ Failure of closed reduction
    - ▪ Middle column injury (PLL, posterior annulus fibrosis)
    - ▪ Associated fractures result in instability
    - ▪ Flexion-extension views demonstrate instability after 12 weeks

## History

► Trauma

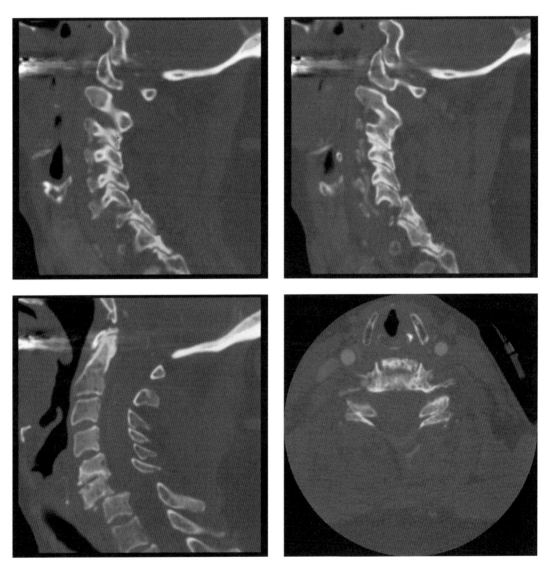

**Figures 23.1–23.4**

# Case 23  Bilateral Facet Dislocation

## Findings

### Radiography

▶ Increased interspinous distance on anteroposterior radiograph = increased space between spinous processes of affected level.

▶ Marked anterior subluxation and prevertebral soft tissue swelling on lateral radiograph.

### CT

▶ Naked facet or "empty hamburger" sign on axial images with uncovered articulating processes.

▶ Marked anterior subluxation of superior vertebral body (in this case C6 on C7), greater than 50% anterolisthesis.

▶ Bilateral jumped or locked facets (inferior articular process lies anterior to the superior articular process on both sides of the spine).

▶ Associated with fractures of the superior facet, inferior facet, and floating lateral mass.

### MRI

▶ Marked anterior subluxation; spinal cord injury including cord edema, hemorrhage, or transection; traumatic disk herniation; and associated ligamentous and paraspinal injury.

## Differential Diagnosis

▶ Unilateral facet dislocation

▶ Facet subluxation

▶ Perched facets

## Teaching Points

▶ Severe unstable hyperflexion distraction injury causing facet joints to jump over each other and become locked.

▶ Disruption of all three spinal columns including all major spinal ligaments, intervertebral disks, and facet joint capsules at the affected level.

▶ Greater than 50% anterior subluxation.

▶ Facets may not dislocate completely and may become perched atop the subjacent facets.

▶ Commonly present with neurologic deficits.

## Management

▶ Operative stabilization and fusion required after reduction because of extensive ligamentous disruption.

### Further Readings

Goldberg AL, Kershah SM. Advances in imaging of vertebral and spinal cord injury. *J Spinal Cord Med.* 2010l;33(2):105–116.

Mhuircheartaigh NN, Kerr JM, Murray JG. MR imaging of traumatic spinal injuries. *Semin Musculoskelet Radiol.* 2006;10(4):293–307.

## History

▶ None

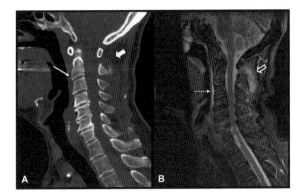

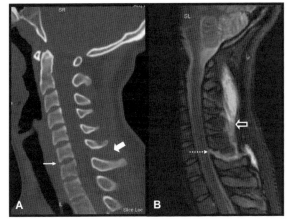

**Figures 24.1–24.2**

# Case 24   Hyperflexion Sprain Injury

## Types

Figure 24.1. C2-3 Hyperflexion Injury. (A) Sagittal image from a non-contrast enhanced cervical spine CT demonstrates a chip fracture of the anteroinferior corner of the C2 vertebral body (thin solid arrow) and fat stranding in the posterior soft tissues suggestive of edema and/or hemorrhage (thick solid arrow). (B) Sagittal STIR image from a non-contrast enhanced cervical spine MRI demonstrates abnormal increased STIR hyperintensity in the anterior (dashed arrow) and posterior (open arrow) soft tissues consistent with soft tissue injury.

Figure 24.2. C6-7 Hyperflexion Injury. (A) Sagittal image from a non-contrast enhanced cervical spine CT demonstrates subtle findings including narrowing of the anterior disc space at the C6-7 level (thin solid arrow), minimal C7 vertebral body height loss and widening of the posterior interspinous space (thick solid arrow). (B) Sagittal STIR image from a non-contrast enhanced cervical spine MRI demonstrates abnormal increased STIR hyperintensity in the posterior soft tissues from C1-C7 particularly in the C6-7 interspinous space (open arrow) and apparent focal rupture of the ligamentum flavum at the C6-7 level (dashed arrow).

Flexion-type injuries of the cervical spine represent a spectrum of injuries bound by a common injury mechanism. Commonly recognized types (in increasing severity) include

- Hyperflexion ligamentous sprain or partial tear
- Clay-shoveler's fracture
- Stable and unstable wedge fracture
- Unilateral facet dislocation
- Bilateral facet dislocation
- Flexion teardrop fracture

Hyperflexion sprain injuries encompass soft tissue injuries of the cervical spine with or without fracture.

## Findings

### Radiograph and CT

- Anterior disk space narrowing and posterior interspinous space widening.
- Translation at the level of ligamentous injury.
- Prominence of the prevertebral soft tissues.

### MRI

- Increased T2-signal involving the spinal ligaments and adjacent soft tissue, most commonly the interspinous ligaments and posterior soft tissues, representing edema and/or hemorrhage.
- Increased T2 or STIR signal involving the anterior portion of the vertebral bodies of the involved level, representing marrow edema secondary to bony contusion.

## Teaching Points

### Etiology

- Hyperflexion is the most common injury mechanism of the cervical spine, accounting for almost half of all cervical spine injuries.
- Eliciting the mechanism of injury and vertebral levels of point tenderness, if available, are of critical importance in identifying subtle injuries.

## Management

Optimal management of unstable injuries or injuries with associated neurologic deficits requires early consultation with a spine surgeon or neurosurgeon. May require early surgical intervention or decompression in the case of spinal cord impingement. Studies evaluating early corticosteroid treatment for neurologic impairment have shown mixed results.

## History

▶ 59-year-old female status post fall down stairs.

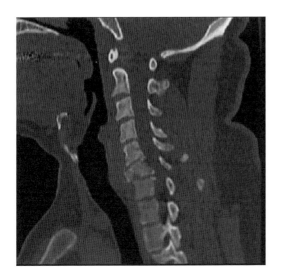 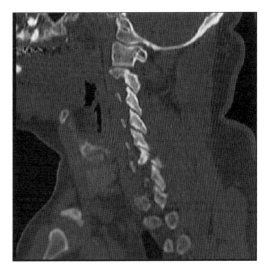

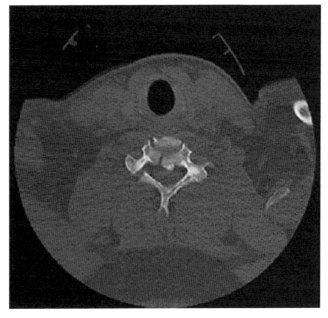

**Figures 25.1–25.3**

# Case 25   Cervical Flexion Teardrop Fracture

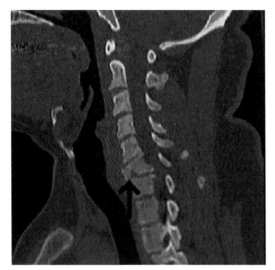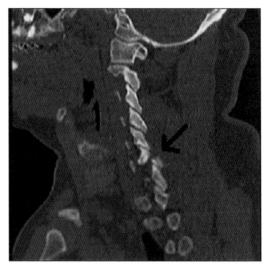

**Figures 25.4–25.5**

## Findings

▶ Figure 25.1. Sagittal view demonstrates anterior greater than posterior compression deformity of the C6 vertebral body.

▶ Figure 25.2. Sagittal view, off midline demonstrates displaced fracture of the facet resulting in facet malalignment.

▶ Figure 25.3. Vertebral body fracture and displaced fracture of the right facet.

▶ Figure 25.4. Arrow denotes the teardrop fracture.

▶ Figure 25.5. Arrow denotes facet fracture.

## Differential Diagnosis

Burst fracture

## Teaching Points

▶ Mechanism: Forceful flexion and axial compression of the cervical spine that occurs when the neck is flexed and the head strikes a solid object, such as in diving into shallow pool of water or hitting head on dashboard in a motor vehicle collision.

▶ Neurologic impact includes anterior cord syndrome: quadraplegia with loss of anterior column senses of pain, temperature, and touch sensations; and preservation of posterior column senses of position, motion, and vibration.

▶ CT and radiographic findings
  ▪ Anteroinferior margin of cervical vertebral body is fractured.
  ▪ Posterior ligaments are disrupted with portion of the vertebral displaced backward into the spinal canal.
  ▪ Intervertebral disk between fractured vertebral body and vertebral body below may be disrupted.
  ▪ Reciprocal distractive force may results in disruption of the posterior structures including the interspinous ligamentous fracture, facet misalignment, and laminar fractures

## Management

Neurosurgical intervention is likely necessary.

### Further Reading

Kim K, Chen H, Russell E, Rogers L. Flexion teardrop fracture of the cervical spine: radiographic characteristics. *Am J Radiol.* 1989;152:319–326.

## History

▶ 48-year-old male construction worker who fell from scaffolding.

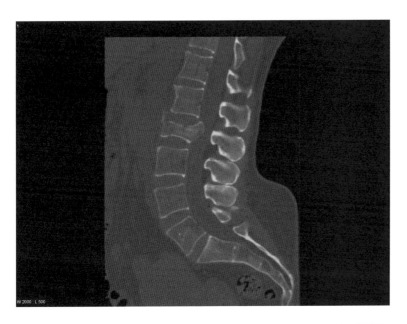

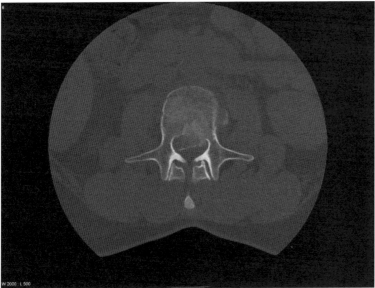

**Figures 26.1–26.2**

# Case 26  Lumbar Burst Fracture

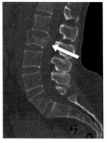 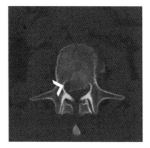

**Figures 26.3–26.4**

## Findings

### Radiograph

▶ Classically demonstrates increased interpedicular distance compared with vertebral body above and below.

### CT

▶ Compression of L2 vertebral body.
▶ Loss of height of posterior cortex with extension of fracture line through it (arrow).
▶ Retropulsion of bone fragment with narrowing of spinal canal (arrowhead).

### Differential Diagnosis

▶ Wedge compression fracture
▶ Split compression fracture
▶ Chance fracture
▶ Pathologic fracture

## Teaching Points

### Etiology

▶ Fall from height with landing on feet is a common mechanism.
▶ Axial loading of vertebral body with compressive failure of anterior and posterior cortex of vertebral body.
▶ Failure of both anterior and middle columns.
▶ With rapid axial load, fluid in nucleus pulposus becomes pressurized and expands in all directions, unable to escape through normal pores and fissures, resulting in bursting of vertebral body as one proposed mechanism.

### Differentiation

▶ Wedge compression and split fractures result from an axial load with a flexion component and failure of the anterior column. The latter is associated with coronal fracture lines through the vertebral body. The posterior cortex is intact with no retropulsion in these types of fractures.
▶ A Chance fracture is a flexion/distraction injury, with anterior wedge compression of the vertebral body and a transverse fracture extending through the posterior elements. This results in compression of the anterior column and distraction of the middle and posterior columns.

### Associations

▶ Lower extremity fractures, pelvic fractures, other spinal fractures, dural laceration, epidural hematoma.

### Management

▶ Conservative if neurologically intact.
▶ Fixation with laminectomy if neurologic deficit, kyphosis >20 degrees, >50% compression of vertebral body, subluxation of facet joints.

### Further Readings

Rutherford EE. Lumbar spine fusion and stabilization: hardware, techniques, and imaging appearances. *Radiographics.* 2007;27:1737–1749.
Heary RF. Decision-making in burst fractures of the thoracolumbar and lumbar spine. *Indian J Orthop.* 2007;41(4): 268–276.

## History

▸ None

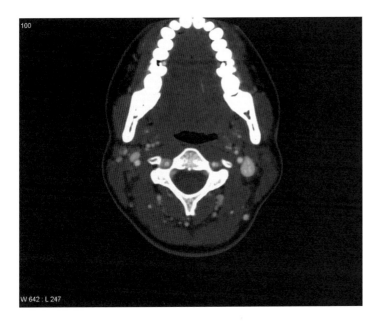

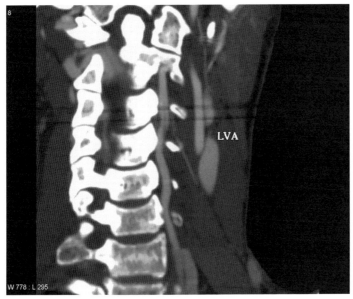

**Figures 27.1–27.2**

# Case 27   Vertebral / Carotid Artery Dissection

## Findings

- Ultrasound: intimal flap, double lumen each with different signal on Doppler flow, dissecting aneurysm
- CT: narrowed lumen, double lumen, dissection flap, hematoma
- MRA: vessel narrowing +/- aneurismal dilation of dissected artery. Susceptibility MR may show blooming artifact of blood products.
- Angiography: gold standard; intimal flap and double lumen; long segment of arterial narrowing "string sign"

## Differential Diagnosis

- Intramural thrombus
- Atheromatous plaque
- Fibromuscular dysplasia
- Pseudoaneurysm
- Glomus vagale paraganglioma
- Carotid space schwannoma

## Teaching Points

- Most frequent presentation is headache. May also experience pain in face or neck, Horner syndrome, brain ischemia, dizziness.
- ICA dissection in young patients, usually at the base of the skull.
- ICA dissection in older patients, usually at the carotid bifurcation.
- Trauma is most common cause.

## Management

- Anticoagulation to prevent thrombosis and embolism in extracranial dissections. Anticoagulation contraindicated in cases of intracranial dissecting aneurysms with subarachnoid hemorrhage.
- Consider endovascular or surgical intervention if persistent symptoms caused by thromboembolic events and/ or dissecting aneurysm.

### Further Readings

Rodallec MH, Marteau V, Gerber S, et al. Craniocervical arterial dissection: spectrum of imaging findings and differential diagnosis. *Radiographics*. 2008;28:1711–1728.

Shin JH, Suh DC, Choi CG, et al. Vertebral artery dissection: spectrum of imaging findings with emphasis on angiography and correlation with clinical presentation. *Radiographics*. 2000;20:1687–1696.

Case 28

## History

► 77-year-old woman with facial and forehead trauma during fall while ambulating.

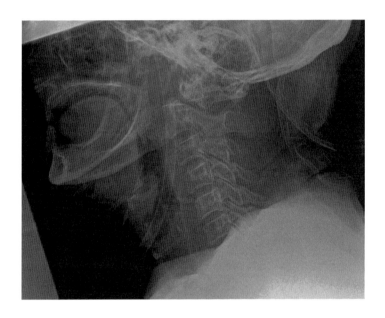

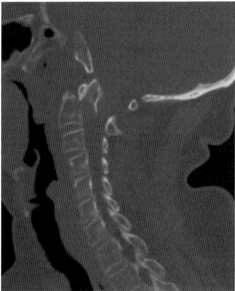

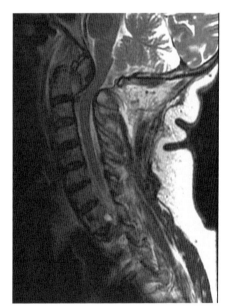

**Figures 28.1–28.3**

Case 28

## History

► 77-year-old woman with facial and forehead trauma during fall while ambulating.

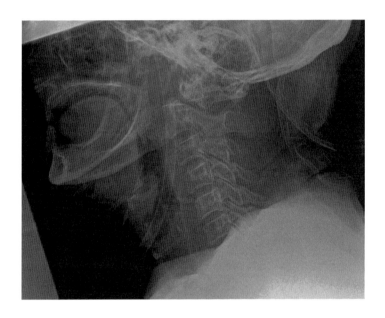

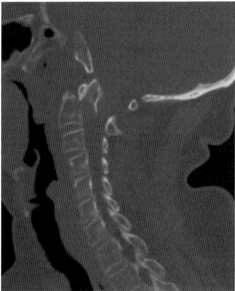

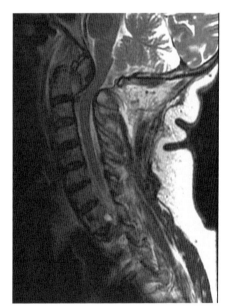

**Figures 28.1–28.3**

61

# Case 28 Odontoid Fracture

**Findings**

▶ Fracture of odontoid process (dens) of the C2 vertebral body.
  ▪ Transverse fracture of dens (type II) with posterior angulation and displacement of proximal fragment. Spinal canal stenosis with cord edema.
▶ Subtypes: (Anderson and D'Alonzo classification).
  ▪ Type I: avulsion fracture through the superolateral extent of odontoid process at attachment of alar ligament (rare).
  ▪ Type II: fracture through junction of odontoid process and body.
    ▪ Increased risk of nonunion (look for these!)
    ▪ Comminution at base of odontoid fracture fragment
    ▪ >5 mm initial translocation
      ▪ Posterior displacement greater risk than anterior
    ▪ >10 degrees angulation
    ▪ Elderly
    ▪ Delayed diagnosis
  ▪ Type III: fracture involving the odontoid process and body of C2.

**Differential Diagnosis**

▶ Os odontoideum
▶ C1/C2 subluxation from ligamentous laxity
  ▪ Rheumatoid arthritis
  ▪ Trisomy 21
▶ Condylus tertius
  ▪ Congenital variant third occipital condyle extending from clivus
▶ Nonfusion of apical odontoid epiphysis (ossiculum terminale)

**Teaching Points**

▶ Etiology
  ▪ Hyperextension or less likely hyperflexion of upper cervical spine
▶ Cord injury rare because of capacious central canal at C1 and C2 levels.
  ▪ Cord injury may occur with severe hyperextension and posterior displacement of coronoid fragment.
▶ Risk of vertebral artery injury if fracture extends through foramen transversarium

**Management**

**Type I**

▶ Most are stable fractures
  ▪ High rate of successful healing with nonoperative treatment
  ▪ Treat with semirigid collar for symptoms
▶ Unstable if flexion/extension reveals subluxation of C1
  ▪ Needs surgical fixation
▶ Unstable if associated with occipitoatlantal dislocation
  ▪ Needs surgical fixation

**Type II**

▶ Unstable; risk of nonunion 30%–50%
▶ Initial management with halo vest
▶ If nonsurgical management fails: surgical fixation

**Type III**

▶ Unstable fracture (occiput, C1, and proximal C2 fragment move as unit increasing motion at fracture site)
▶ High rate of successful healing with nonoperative treatment

# Section 3    Chest

**History**

► None

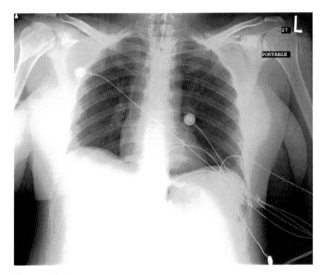

**Figure 29.1**

# Case 29   Occult Pneumothorax

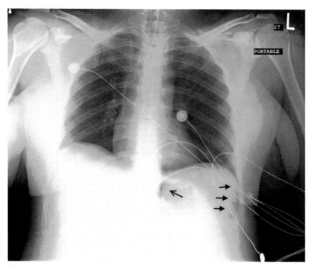

**Figure 29.2**

## Findings

▶ Hyperlucent left upper quadrant
▶ Widening and deepening of the left costophrenic angle (solid arrow)
▶ Triangular lucency medial left cardiophrenic sulcus (open arrow)

## Differential Diagnosis

▶ Normal
▶ Skin fold
▶ External artifact: sheets, clothing, hair braids
▶ Bullous disease
▶ Pneumoperitoneum

## Teaching Points

▶ Identification of a pneumothorax on plain radiography relies primarily on visualization of the pleural line between the aerated lung and the pathologically air-filled potential space of the pleura. Thus, if the pleural edge is not tangential to the X-ray beam, a pleural line is not necessarily seen. This is particularly true in the supine radiograph.
▶ Most common locations: anteromedial, subpulmonic, apicolateral, posteromedial
▶ Deep sulcus sign: larger/wider lateral costophrenic recess than contralateral side
▶ Hyperlucent upper abdominal quadrant
▶ Outline of the medial diaphragm beneath the cardiac silhouette
▶ Sharply defined diaphragmatic contour despite dense lung parenchymal air space disease

## Management

▶ Cross-sectional imaging may be needed for confirmation
▶ Pneumothoraces normally resorb at ~1% per day
▶ Thoracotomy tube may be necessary if clinically symptomatic

## Further Readings

Tocino I. Pneumothorax in the supine patient: radiographic anatomy. *RadioGraphics*. 1985;5(4):557–586.
McLoud TC, Boiselle PM. *Thoracic Radiology: The Requisites*. 2nd ed. Philadelphia: Mosby Elsevier; 2010:422.

## History

▸ 55-year-old female with the acute onset of chest pain.

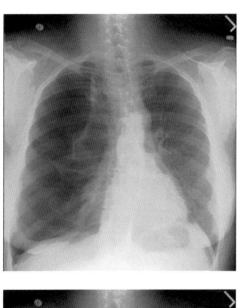
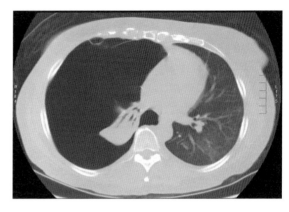
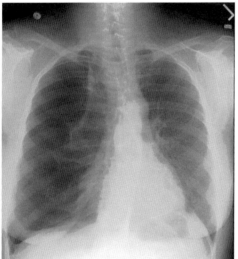
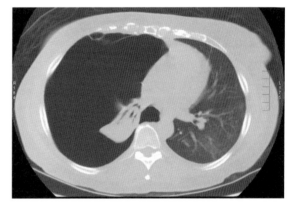

**Figures 30.1–30.4**

# Case 30  Tension Pneumothorax

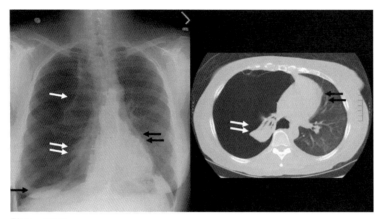

**Figure 30.5**

## Findings

▶ Frontal radiograph of the chest and axial image from a subsequent chest CT (Figure 30.5) demonstrate a sharp right pleural line without lung markings seen in the lung periphery (white arrow).

▶ The right lung is collapsed (double white arrows).

▶ There is flattening of the right hemidiaphragm (black arrow) and shifting of the mediastinum to the left (double black arrows), suggestive of tension.

## Differential Diagnosis

▶ Spontaneous
▶ Traumatic
▶ Iatrogenic
▶ COPD
▶ Interstitial lung diseases, such as lymphangiomyomatosis
▶ Infectious
▶ Connective tissue disorders

## Teaching Points

▶ Tension pneumothorax has severe consequences, including death, if left untreated.

▶ Radiographic signs of pneumothorax include a sharp pleural line with an absence of lung markings distally, hyperlucent lung, hyperlucent upper abdominal quadrants, and a deep costophrenic sulcus.

▶ Radiographic signs of tension pneumothorax include splaying of the ribs on the side of pneumothorax, shifting of the mediastinum away from the pneumothorax, and ipsilateral flattening of the hemidiaphragm.

▶ Tension pneumothorax is easily treated with needle decompression, thus prompt recognition and communication of this diagnosis to the referring physician is essential. Documentation of this emergent communication should be included in the radiology report along with the method of communication, the time the communication took place, and the name of physician who received the communication.

## Management

▶ Needle decompression
▶ Emergent communication with the referring physician by the interpreting physician

## Further Readings

Leigh-Smith S, Harris T. Tension pneumothorax—time for a re-think? *Emerg Med J.* 2005;22(8):8–16.
American College of Radiology Practice Guideline for Communication of Diagnostic Imaging Findings. Revised 2010. Downloaded from http://www.acr.org/secondarymainmenucategories/quality_safety/guidelines/dx/comm_diag_rad.aspx on 2/21/12

## History

▶ None

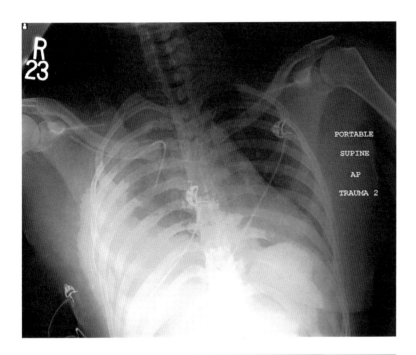

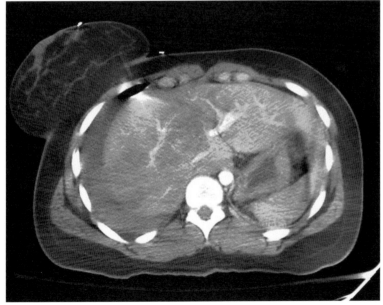

**Figures 31.1–31.2**

# Case 31  Hemothorax

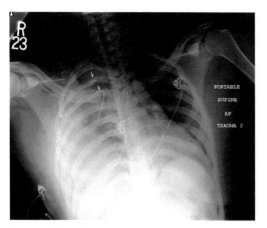 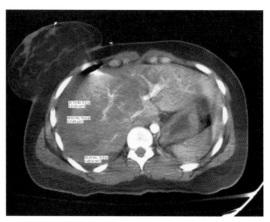

**Figures 31.3–31.4**

## Findings
### Plain Film
▶ Right-sided pleural effusion and air space opacity
▶ Multiple right-sided rib fractures

### Computed Tomography
▶ Hyperdense fluid (blood) contained within the pleural space
▶ Regions of interest demonstrate increasing density with dependency

## Differential Diagnosis
▶ Pleural effusion
▶ Chylothorax
▶ Pleural-based mass/scarring

## Teaching Points
▶ Although most commonly associated with chest wall trauma, it can be seen with thoracic aortic injury, anticoagulation, metastatic malignancy, tuberculosis, and pulmonary infarct.
▶ A single hemithorax can hold 4 L of blood, allowing for exsanguination.
▶ Blood tends to clot quickly followed by a decrease in density with evolution and lysis.
▶ Empyema can develop if it becomes superinfected.
▶ Fibrothorax can develop from fibrous adhesions. This can yield scarring and even entrapment of the underlying lung.

## Management
▶ Generally treated with single or double thoracotomy tubes depending on size (proper positioning should be inferior and posterior for fluid, compared with apical and anterior for air)
▶ Surgical intervention may be required if there is immediate removal of >1 L of acute hemorrhage or if there is continued bleeding >200 cc/h over 2–4 hours
▶ If large clot persists (i.e., retained hemothorax >500 cc), chemical lysis with fibrinolytic agents may be used to decrease the risk of empyema or fibrothoroax development

## Further Readings

Chest trauma hemothorax. *Trauma.org*. http://www.trauma.org/archive/thoracic/CHESThaemo.html.
McLoud TC, Boiselle PM. *Thoracic Radiology: The Requisites*. 2nd ed. Philadelphia: Mosby Elsevier; 2010:422.
Parry GW, Morgan WE, Salama FD. Management of haemothorax. *Ann R Coll Surg Engl*. 1996;78:325–326.

**History**

▶ None

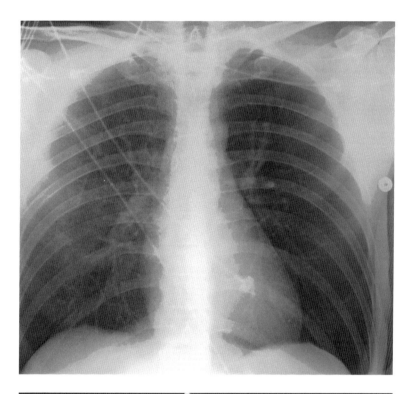

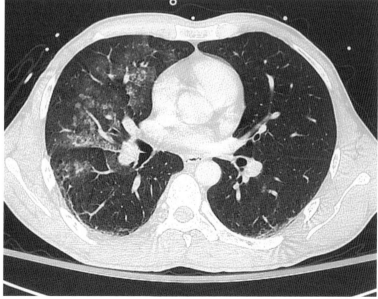

**Figures 32.1–32.2**

# Case 32 Pulmonary Contusion

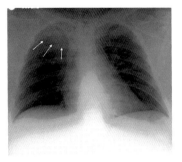 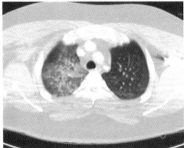 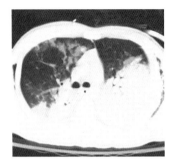

**Figures 32.3–32.5**

## Findings

▶ Chest radiograph: Vague opacity right mid lung
▶ CT: Patchy alveolar and ground-glass opacities throughout the right lung
▶ Additional images from different patients demonstrate similar findings in the right upper lobe (Figures 32.3, 32.4), and patchy RML contusions and more dense posterior contusions in a separate patient (Figure 32.5)

## Differential Diagnosis

▶ Other air space processes: Pneumonia, aspiration, edema, ARDS

## Teaching Points

▶ Pulmonary contusion is one of the most common findings in blunt chest trauma
  ▪ They are the most common chest injury in children
▶ Etiology is from traumatic hemorrhage into the lung parenchyma and air spaces
▶ Although up to one-third are inapparent on initial radiography, they generally become apparent within 6 hours of initiating trauma, and almost always by 24 hours
▶ Clinical symptoms range from clinically silent to hemoptysis and impaired gas exchange
▶ Radiographically appears the same as any other air space process
  ▪ Alveolar filling can yield ground-glass or "fluffy" infiltrates to dense consolidation
  ▪ May or may not demonstrate air bronchograms secondary to bronchial filling with hemorrhage
  ▪ Can be contralateral to side of injury (contrecoup)
▶ Look for associated blunt force injury (i.e., rib fractures, flail chest, scapular fractures, soft tissue contusions)

## Management

▶ If small, can resolve rapidly (often within 24–48 hours), but most resolve with 3–5 days.
▶ More advanced disease can lead to impaired oxygenation, increased pulmonary vascular resistance, and decreased lung compliance.
▶ 40% of patients require mechanical ventilation, 50%–60% of severe contusions develop bilateral acute respiratory distress syndrome (ARDS).
▶ Clinical management involves fluid restriction; however, this must be weighted with the risk of hypoperfusion, which is associated with development of ARDS in addition to multiorgan consequences.
▶ Most frequent complication is pneumonia.

### Further Readings

Brohi K. Chest trauma pulmonary contusion. *Trauma.org.* http://www.trauma.org/archive/thoracic/CHESTcontusion.
Wagner RB. Classification of parenchymal injuries of the lung. *Radiology.* 1988;167:77–82.

## History

▶ 23-year-old female status post high-impact motor vehicle accident with left-sided chest pain.

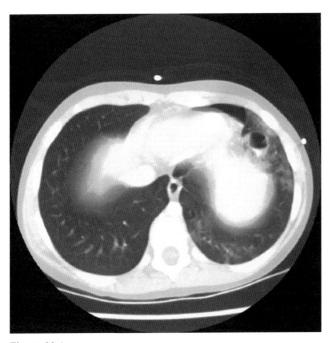

**Figure 33.1**

# Case 33  Lung Laceration

## Findings

▶ Axial CT image demonstrates a cavitary rounded lesion with air-fluid level consistent with lung laceration. Of note, there is adjacent lung contusion and small pneumothorax.

## Differential Diagnosis

▶ Pneumatocele
▶ Lung laceration otherwise has a fairly pathognomic appearance. If not provided history of acute injury, CT or radiographic findings could also be similar to those of
  ▪ Cavitary malignant nodule
  ▪ Cavitary infection/nodule

## Teaching Points

▶ Pulmonary lacerations result from both blunt and penetrating trauma
▶ Can be a marker for high-energy mechanism of injury
▶ Can be associated with lung contusion, pneumothorax, or hemothorax
▶ Complications not common but can include infection, abscess, pneumothorax, or bronchopleural fistula formation
▶ CT is more sensitive than chest radiography
▶ Imaging signs of lung laceration include round or ovoid structures that can be filled with either air, hemorrhage, or other fluid; air-fluid levels may be present; multiple lacerations may be present

## Management

▶ Most commonly, expectant management unless there are complications
▶ If complications or if severe laceration, surgical treatment including suturing, stapling, and wedge resection can be considered

### Further Readings

Kaewlai R, Avery LL, Asrani AV, et al. Multidetector CT of blunt thoracic trauma. *RadioGraphics*. 2008;28(6):1555–1570.
Hollister M, Stern EJ, Steinberg KP. Type 2 pulmonary laceration: a marker of blunt high-energy injury to the lung. *AJR Am J Roentgenol*. 1995;165(5):1126.

## History

▸ 34-year-old male status post high-impact front-end motor vehicle accident found to have tracheal injury via CT and confirmed diagnosis via bronchoscopy.

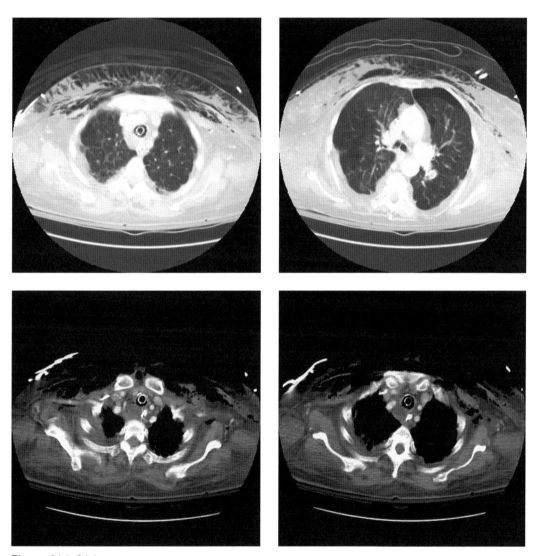

**Figures 34.1–34.4**

# Case 34 Tracheobronchial Injury

### Findings

▶ Axial CT images in lung windows (Figure 34.1) demonstrate extensive subcutaneous emphysema and concurrent pneumothorax indicating high-impact mechanism of injury (Figure 34.2).

▶ Axial CT image (Figure 34.3) in mediastinal windows demonstrates posterior wall irregularity and caliber increase of trachea with small foci of extraluminal mediastinal air adjacent to the right of trachea (Figure 34.4).

### Differential Diagnosis of Tracheal Rupture

▶ Tracheal diverticulum
▶ Tracheoesophageal fistula
▶ Pneumomediastinum

### Teaching Points

▶ Radiographic findings: Tracheal dilatation, pneumomediastinum, or subcutaneous emphysema.
▶ CT findings: Abrupt dilatation and increase in caliber of diameter of trachea, adjacent pneumomediastinum, mediastinal hematoma, or tracheal wall irregularity or outpouching.
▶ Associated imaging findings: Extensive subcutaneous emphysema, pneumothorax, or other associated chest wall trauma.
▶ Chest radiographs are not sensitive when compared with CT in detecting tracheal injury.

### Management

▶ Dependent on location and severity of the injury and if patient is stable.
▶ Goal of treatment is to ensure a patent airway to prevent respiratory compromise.
▶ Intubation and mechanical ventilation is initial first-line treatment.
▶ Consideration of laryngoscopy and bronchoscopy for further evaluation.
▶ Although less severe cases can be managed without surgery, surgical intervention is considered the gold standard for treatment of any tracheal or bronchial tear.

### Further Readings

Kaewlai R, Avery LL, Asrani AV, et al. Multidetector CT of blunt thoracic trauma. *RadioGraphics*. 2008;28(6):1555–1570.

Chen JD, Shanmuganathan K, Mirvis SE, Killeen KL, Dutton RP. Using CT to diagnose tracheal rupture. *AJR Am J Roentgenol*. 2001;176(5):1273–1280.

## History

▶ 35-year-old male status post front-end motor vehicle accident

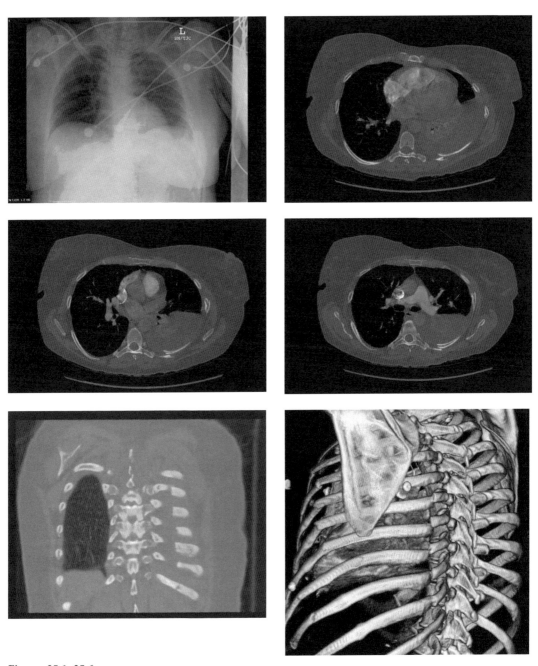

**Figures 35.1–35.6**

# Case 35   Flail Chest

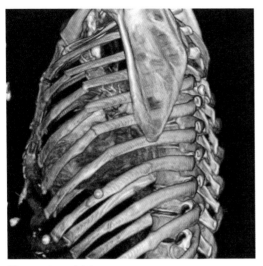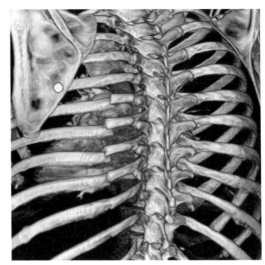

**Figures 35.7–35.8**

## Findings

▶ Frontal radiograph of the chest (Figure 35.1) demonstrates multiple left-sided rib fractures.
▶ CT image (Figures 35.2, 35.3, 35.4, 35.5) shows multiple ribs (>3) with fractures in two or more locations.
▶ Three-dimensional volume rendering (Figures 35.6, 35.7, 35.8) illustrates multiple ribs (>3) with fractures in two or more locations.

## Differential Diagnosis

▶ If meeting definition of three or more ribs fractured in two or more locations, flail chest has a fairly characteristic appearance.

## Teaching Points

▶ Flail chest is usually associated with high-impact mechanisms of blunt trauma.
▶ Flail chest is essentially segment of thoracic ribs being separated from remainder of chest wall.
▶ Can be life-threatening given high association with other injuries.
▶ If a patient presents with flail chest, there are usually additional associated injuries, such as pneumothorax, hemothorax, lung laceration, or lung contusions.
▶ Clinical examination reveals a paradoxical movement of the flail segment during breathing.
▶ Radiographic findings: Flail chest occurs when three or more ribs are fractured in two or more locations.
▶ Chest radiographs are not as sensitive as CT in clearly defining flail segments.

## Management

▶ Critical care including mechanical ventilation and close monitoring
▶ Surgical treatment is required in severe cases and can result in faster ventilator wean time, and shorter ICU stay

## Further Readings

Pettiford BL, Luketich JD, Landreneau RJ. The management of flail chest. *Thorac Surg Clin.* 2007;17(1):25–33.
Collins J. Chest wall trauma. *J Thorac Imaging.* 2000;15(2):112–119.

## History

▸ 65-year-old man who was the unrestrained driver in a motor vehicle collision

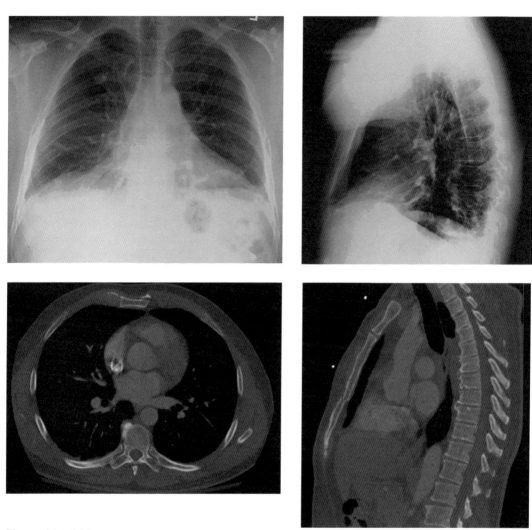

**Figures 36.1–36.4**

# Case 36  Sternal Fracture

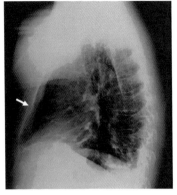 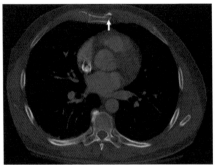 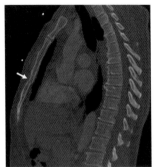

**Figures 36.5–36.7**

## Findings

▶ Lateral (Figure 36.5) radiograph of the chest demonstrate a fracture of the mid-sternum (arrow) with some anterior displacement of the distal fracture fragment. This finding is confirmed on axial (Figure 36.6) and sagittal reformatted (Figure 36.7) images from contrast-enhanced chest CT in bone windows (arrow).

## Differential Diagnosis

▶ Pectus excavatum
▶ Pathologic fracture
▶ Osteomyelitis
▶ Ossification center

## Teaching Points

▶ Sternal fractures are most commonly the result of motor vehicle collisions with deceleration injury to the chest.
▶ CT is the modality of choice to evaluate for sternal fractures, which are best demonstrated on sagittally reformatted images.
▶ Sternal fractures can be subtle and are frequently nondisplaced. Often, the only clue to the presence of a sternal fracture is a mediastinal hematoma
▶ Mediastinal hematomas from sternal fracture can be distinguished from those associated with aortic injury by the presence of a fat plane between the hematoma and the aorta
▶ Sternal fractures are associated with high-energy trauma; thus, careful evaluation for injury to the heart and aorta is warranted.

## Management

▶ Careful evaluation for other injuries in the chest, especially to the heart and aorta
▶ Adequate analgesia with possible surgical intervention

## History

▶ 41-year-old male status post front-end motor vehicle accident with air-bag deployment presenting with chest pain.

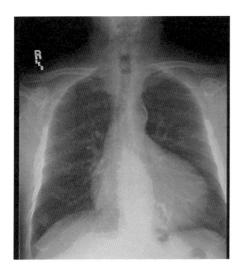
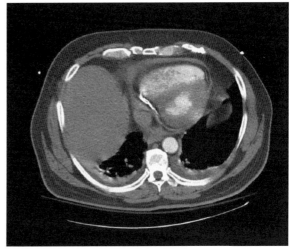
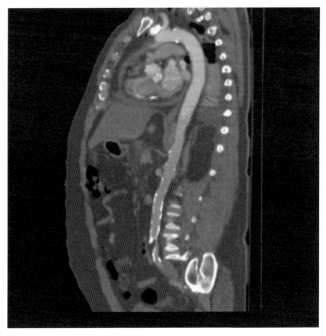

**Figures 37.1–37.3**

# Case 37  Hemopericardium in Blunt Cardiac Trauma (Myocardial Injury)

## Findings

▶ Frontal radiograph of the chest (Figure 37.1) demonstrates an enlarged cardiac silhouette.

▶ Axial (Figure 37.2) and sagittal (Figure 37.3) CT images demonstrate a hyperdense pericardial effusion consistent with hemopericardium. Of note, no aortic dissection is present raising concern for hemopericardium from underlying myocardial injury.

## Differential Diagnosis

▶ Inflammatory pericardial effusion
▶ Infected pericardial effusion
▶ Aortic dissection resulting in hemopericardium

## Teaching Points

▶ Hemopericardium can occur secondary to occult myocardial muscle injury, such as from infarct or direct tissue injury. However, although not as common, hemopericardium can also occur in setting of myocardial rupture.

▶ Hemopericardium can also occur in setting of ascending aortic dissection. Hence, it is important to evaluate and exclude associated traumatic aortic injury in trauma patients.

▶ Radiographic findings: Enlarged cardiac silhouette suggestive of a pericardial effusion.

▶ CT findings: Hemopericardium appears as a hyperdense pericardial effusion.

▶ Cardiac tamponade is a life-threatening condition that can result from hemopericardium; cardiac tamponade is a clinical diagnosis but imaging may provide early warning.

▶ Can be associated with constrictive pericarditis and may be delayed in nature because of evolution of myocardial muscle contusion and/or infarction.

▶ Close interval and continuous monitoring after presentation is required to evaluate for cardiac tamponade.

## Management

▶ Close monitoring for worsening of hemopericardium and to detect cardiac tamponade.
▶ If necessary, surgical treatment and drainage of pericardial effusion.

### Further Readings

Krejci CS, Blackmore CC, Nathens A. Hemopericardium: an emergent finding in a case of blunt cardiac injury. *AJR Am J Roentgenol.* 2000 Jul;175(1):250.

Pretre R, Chilcott M. Blunt trauma to the heart and great vessels. *N Engl J Med.* 1997;336(9):626–632.

Goldstein L, Mirvis SE, Kostrubiak IS, Turney SZ. CT diagnosis of acute pericardial tamponade after blunt chest trauma. *AJR Am J Roentgenol.* 1989 Apr;152(4):739–41.

## History

▶ None

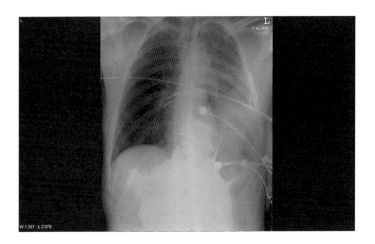

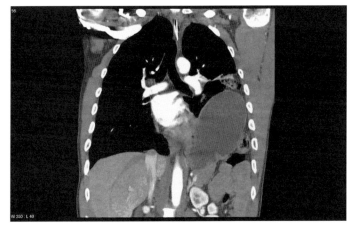

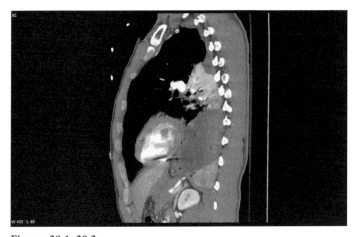

**Figures 38.1–38.3**

# Case 38   Diaphragmatic Rupture

**Findings**

**Plain Film**

- ▶ Elevated hemidiaphragm
- ▶ Hemithorax opacity
- ▶ Mediastinal shift to nonaffected side
- ▶ Presence of traumatic thoracic injuries (rib fractures, pneumothorax, and so forth).

**CT**

- ▶ Diaphragmatic defect with herniation of abdominal contents into the thorax
- ▶ Focal constriction of the herniated contents (collar sign)
- ▶ Dependent location of herniated abdominal contents (dependent viscera sign)

**Differential Diagnosis**

- ▶ Bochdalek or Morgagni hernia
- ▶ Hiatal hernia
- ▶ Eventration of the hemidiaphragm
- ▶ Paralysis of the hemidiaphragm
- ▶ Pleural lesions

**Teaching Points**

- ▶ CT is best modality for evaluation.
- ▶ Most common cause is penetrating trauma from knife/gunshot wounds or blunt trauma from motor vehicle accidents and falls.
- ▶ Rupture from blunt trauma may present years after inciting event.

**Management**

- ▶ Early diagnosis and surgical repair for best prognosis.

Further Readings

Desir A, Ghaye B. CT of blunt diaphragmatic rupture. *Radiographics.* 2012 Mar-Apr;32(2):477–98.

McLoud TC, Boiselle PM. "Thoracic trauma." In: *Thoracic Radiology: The Requisites,* 2e (Requisites in Radiology) Philadelphia, PA: Mosby; 2010. pp. 160–180.

▸ None

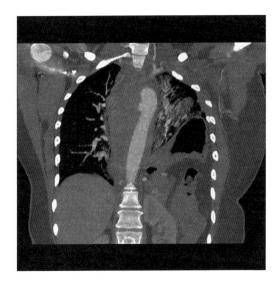 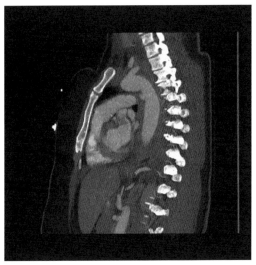

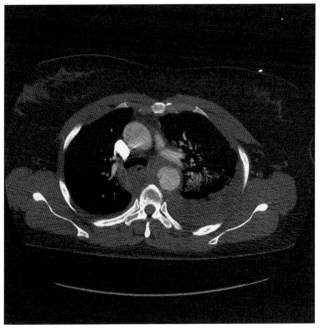

**Figures 39.1–39.3**

# Case 39  Aortic injury

## Findings

▶ Pseudoaneurysm with extensive mediastinal hematoma (Figure 39.1)
▶ Pseudoaneurysm with extensive mediastinal hematoma (Figure 39.2)
▶ Small intimal flap with mediastinal hematoma and left hemothorax and pulmonary contusion (Figure 39.3)

## Teaching Points

▶ Most acute traumatic aortic injuries (ATAI) result from rapid deceleration, most commonly as a result of a motor vehicle collision, especially head-on and side-impact collisions. Proposed mechanisms contributing to ATAI include shearing forces, rapid deceleration, hydrostatic forces, and the osseous pinch.
▶ Immediately lethal in up to 90% of cases with mortality rapidly rising within the first 24 hours if they are left untreated, which underscores the importance of rapid diagnosis and definitive therapy.
▶ Thoracic aortic rupture (TAR) is recognized as a cause of death in victims of blunt trauma.
▶ Immediate mortality is 85% but in the group who survive to reach hospital there is a reasonable chance of successful surgical repair.
▶ Contrast-enhanced CT has been established as the imaging modality of choice for stable patients with a high-risk mechanism of injury and clinical features or chest radiologic abnormalities suggestive of TAR.

## Typical CT findings

▶ Intramural hematoma with or without intimal tear
▶ Abrupt change in aortic caliber
▶ Diminished caliber of the descending aorta (pseudocoarctation)
▶ Pseudoaneurysm
▶ Extravasation of contrast material

The extent and morphology of aortic injuries vary widely, ranging from intimal hemorrhage to complete transection.

Most injuries occur at the junction of the arch and proximal descending thoracic aorta.

Partial lacerations usually involve only the inner two vessel wall layers, resulting in a contained rupture.

Adventitial injuries are almost universally fatal because of rapid exsanguination. Temporary tamponade may be achieved by surrounding mediastinal soft tissues.

## Management

▶ Within the past decade, endovascular therapy has gained increased acceptance, primarily because of a significant decrease in mortality and morbidity compared with those of surgery.
▶ Complications after endovascular repair include endoleak, endograft collapse, stroke, upper extremity ischemia, paraplegia, graft infection, endograft structural failure, missed injury or stent migration, and access site complications.
▶ Complications after surgical repair, paraplegia and ischemia to other organs, graft dehiscence, graft infection, and graft stenosis may occur.

# Section 4    Abdomen

## History

► Trauma

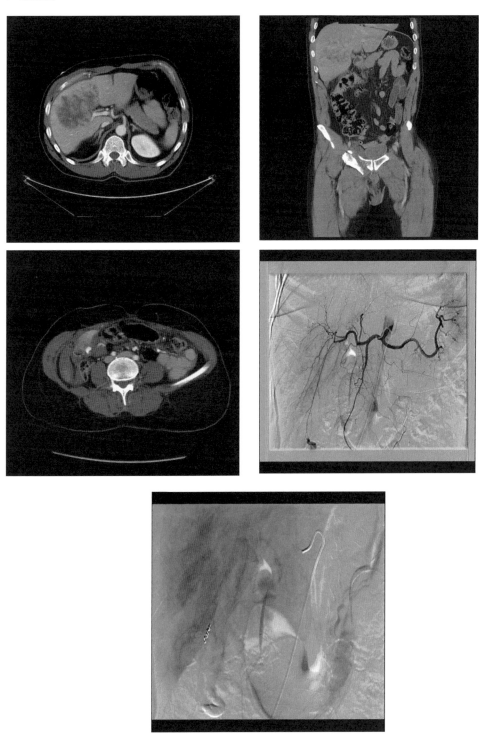

**Figures 40.1–40.5**

# Case 40 Liver Injury

## Findings

▶ Laceration: Irregular linear/branching hypodensities on contrast-enhanced CT indicates tearing of hepatic parenchyma.

▶ Subcapsular hematoma: Oval hypodensity that indents the hepatic contour (as opposed to perihepatic fluid, which does not).

▶ Intraparenchymal hematoma/contusion: Focal, hypodense areas on contrast-enhanced CT, usually with poorly defined margins.

▶ Active hemorrhage: Manifests as extravasation of contrast, either into an intraparenchymal hematoma or into the peritoneal cavity.

▶ Laceration extending into the major hepatic veins or IVC is a particularly concerning feature and usually represents an indication for surgery.

▶ Low-density fluid collections representing bilomas may be seen adjacent to traumatized liver.

## Teaching Points

▶ The liver is the second most frequently injured (20%) intra-abdominal organ, in part because of its relatively fixed position and large size.

▶ Liver laceration is half as frequent as splenic laceration but results in greater morbidity.

▶ AAST grading system
  ▪ Grade I
    ▪ Subcapsular hematoma, <10% surface area
    ▪ Laceration extending <1 cm into parenchyma
  ▪ Grade II
    ▪ Subcapsular hematoma, 10–50% of surface area
    ▪ Intraparenchymal hematoma <10 cm diameter
    ▪ Laceration extending 1–3 cm into parenchyma
  ▪ Grade III
    ▪ Subcapsular hematoma >50% surface area or expanding or ruptured
    ▪ Intraparenchymal hematoma ≥10 cm diameter or expanding or ruptured
    ▪ Laceration >3 cm depth
  ▪ Grade IV
    ▪ Ruptured intraparenchymal hematoma with active bleeding
    ▪ Laceration involving 25–75% of a hepatic lobe or one to three segments of a lobe
  ▪ Grade V
    ▪ Laceration involving >75% of a hepatic lobe of >3 segments of a lobe
    ▪ Involvement of major venous structures (retrohepatic IVC, major hepatic veins)
  ▪ Grade VI
    ▪ Hepatic avulsion

▶ Extension of lacerations into the major hepatic venous structures is correlated with severe injuries, including arterial bleeding, and increased risk for delayed complications.

▶ Periportal low attenuation could represent blood tracking adjacent to portal branches or dilated periportal lymphatics related to elevated central venous pressure.

▶ Intrahepatic or subcapsular gas maybe detected, usually 1–3 days after injury, and may be secondary to either necrosis rather than infection.

## Management

▶ Approximately 80% of traumatic liver injuries are treated nonoperatively.

▶ Active hemorrhage detected with CT may be treated with angiography and embolization.

▶ Biliary endostent placement and percutaneous catheter drainage may be useful in nonsurgical management of complications.

## History

▶ 14-year-old male with abdominal pain and vomiting after a motor vehicle accident.

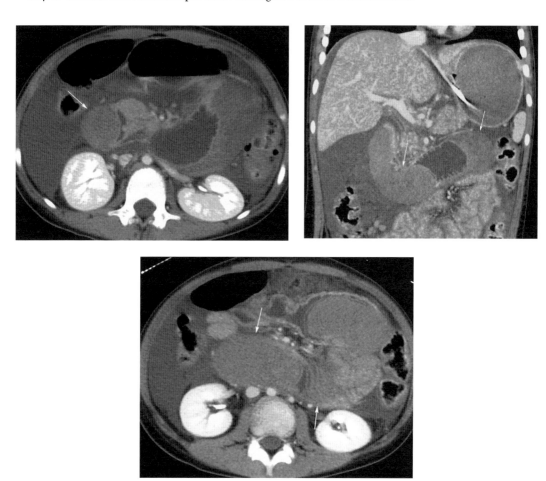

**Figures 41.1–41.3**

# Case 41 Duodenal Hematoma

## Findings

### CT

▶ Eccentric or concentric high density within the duodenal wall (arrows)
▶ Narrowing of the duodenal lumen with upstream gastric dilation depending on the size and extent of hematoma
▶ Free air, wall discontinuity, and/or extraluminal contrast seen with perforation

### Fluoroscopy—Upper GI Series

▶ Narrowing of the duodenal lumen with "coil spring" appearance
▶ Delayed transit of contrast material
▶ Extravasation with perforation

## Differential Diagnosis

▶ Perforated duodenal ulcer
▶ Extensive blood clot within the duodenal lumen from other GI source
▶ Small bowel mass
▶ Crohn disease

## Teaching Points

▶ Mechanism of injury
 ▪ Blunt trauma causing compression of the duodenum against the spinal column (e.g., seat belt injuries, deceleration trauma, sports injuries, and handlebar compression)
 ▪ Nonaccidental trauma should be considered in children <4 years old
▶ Second and third segments are most commonly affected
▶ Commonly associated with injury to the pancreas (coexist in >50% of cases)
▶ Other causes
 ▪ Iatrogenic (e.g., endoscopy, pH probe placement)
 ▪ Bleeding disorders
 ▪ Henoch-Schönlein purpura
▶ AAST grading
 ▪ I: Hematoma of a single segment or partial-thickness laceration
 ▪ II: Hematoma involving multiple segments or laceration with disruption of <50% circumference
 ▪ III: Laceration with disruption of 50%–75% of the circumference of second segment; disruption of 50%–100% of the circumference of any other segment
 ▪ IV: Laceration/disruption of >75% of the circumference of second segment or involvement of the ampulla or common bile duct
 ▪ V: Laceration/massive disruption of the duodenopancreatic complex or duodenal devascularization
 ▪ For multiple injuries, the grade is advanced by one

## Management

▶ Supportive/nonoperative for low-grade, isolated hematomas without perforation
▶ Surgical management for duodenal perforation or significant associated pancreatic injury

## History

▶ Male stabbed with an ice pick and repeated blows to the abdomen. Physical evaluation demonstrated superficial lacerations and ecchymosis along the left flank.

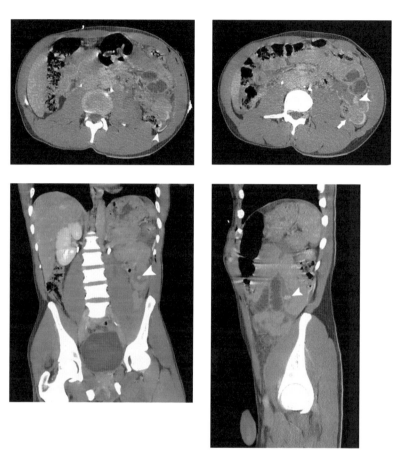

**Figures 42.1–42.4**

# Case 42  Small bowel/Mesenteric Injury

## Findings

- Figures 42.1 and 42.2: Contrast-enhanced CT of the abdomen demonstrates hyperenhancing bowel in the left midabdomen with discontinuous mucosa surrounded by intermediate-density fluid (arrow). Intraluminal focal blush of contrast represents active bleeding that layers dependently in the peritoneum (arrowheads).
- Figures 42.3 and 42.4: Coronal and sagittal reformatted CT images demonstrate a focal hyperattenuating blush in the bowel lumen. Thickened bowel and peritoneal fluid are noted.

## Differential Diagnosis

- Blunt versus penetrating small bowel injury with perforation
- Focal ileus
- Shock bowel
- Ingested material

## Teaching Points

- Abdominopelvic CT is the preferred diagnostic examination for the evaluation of penetrating and blunt abdominal trauma in hemodynamically stable patients.
- Unstable patients should undergo exploratory laparotomy.
- Although the solid organs of the abdomen are more commonly injured, bowel injury represents approximately 5% of blunt abdominal injuries.
- Meticulous and systematic interrogation of the bowel and the use of coronal and sagittal reformatting improve detection rates of bowel injury; however, CT may not be able to pinpoint the exact site of injury.
- CT's accuracy of detecting small bowel injury is 82%, with a sensitivity of 64% and specificity of 97%.
- Findings that suggest bowel injury include focal bowel wall thickening, bowel hematoma, extravasation of contrast into the bowel lumen, focal abnormal wall enhancement, bowel perforation, and intermediate fluid in the dependent peritoneum or retroperitoneum.

## Management

- Small bowel injury represents a small portion of the injuries associated with blunt abdominal trauma.
- Small bowel injury is often noted in association with solid organ injury. In cases of perforation, surgical repair is warranted.
- Less severe cases of bowel hematoma or nonspecific fluid may warrant close monitoring in the context of the patient's overall injury profile.

## Further Readings

LeBedis CA, Anderson SW, Soto JA. CT imaging of blunt traumatic bowel and mesenteric injuries. *Radiol Clin North Am*. 2012;50(1):123–136

Killeen KL, Shanmuganathan K, Poletti PA, et al. Helical computed tomography of bowel and mesenteric injuries. *J Trauma*. 2001;51(1):26–36.

## History

▸ 45-year-old male status post blunt abdominal trauma

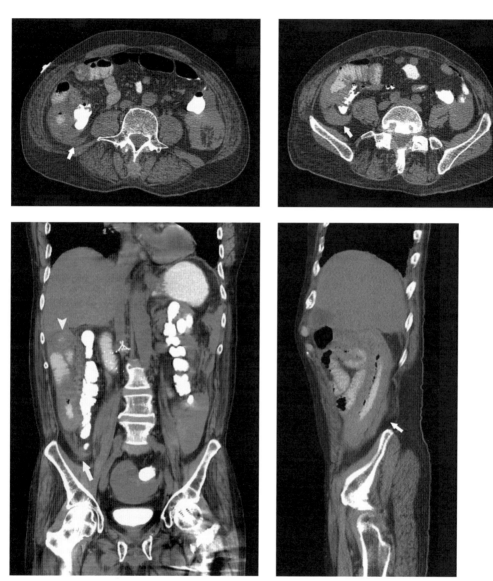

**Figures 43.1–43.4**

# Case 43   Colon Injury

### Findings

▶ Figures 43.1 and 43.2: CT of the abdomen demonstrates thickened ascending and descending colon with intermediate density fluid layering in the paracolonic gutters (arrow).
▶ Figure 43.3: Coronal reformatted image of the abdomen demonstrates a thickened colonic segment (arrow).
▶ Figure 43.4: Sagittal reformatted image of the abdomen demonstrates thickened ascending colon with adjacent intermediate attenuating layering fluid.

### Differential Diagnosis

▶ Blunt traumatic colonic injury
▶ Colitis (infectious, inflammatory, or ischemic)
▶ Colonic hemorrhage

### Teaching Points

▶ Abdominopelvic CT is the preferred diagnostic examination for the evaluation of penetrating and blunt abdominal trauma in hemodynamically stable patients.
▶ Unstable patients should undergo exploratory laparotomy.
▶ Bowel injury represents less than 10% of blunt abdominal injuries.
▶ Meticulous and systematic interrogation of the bowel and the use of coronal and sagittal reformatting improve detection rates of bowel injury; however, CT may not be able to pinpoint the exact site of injury.
▶ CT's accuracy of detecting small bowel injury is 82%, with a sensitivity of 64% and specificity of 97%.
▶ Findings that suggest bowel injury include focal bowel wall thickening, bowel hematoma, extravasation of contrast into the bowel lumen, focal abnormal wall enhancement, bowel perforation, and intermediate fluid in the dependent peritoneum or retroperitoneum.

### Management

▶ Colonic injury represents a small portion of the injuries associated with blunt abdominal trauma.
▶ In cases of perforation, surgical repair is warranted.
▶ Less severe cases of bowel hematoma or nonspecific fluid may warrant close monitoring in the context of the patient's overall injury profile.

### Further Readings

Brasel KJ, Olson CJ, Stafford RE, Johnson TJ. Incidence and significance of free fluid on abdominal computed tomographic scan in blunt trauma. *J Trauma*. 1998;44(5):889–892.
Eanniello VC, Gabram SG, Eusebio R, Jacobs LM. Isolated free fluid on abdominal computerized tomographic scan: an indication for surgery in blunt trauma patients? *Connecticut Medicine*. 1994;58(12):707–710.

## History

▸ 25-year-old male with abdominal pain and nausea following an MVA.

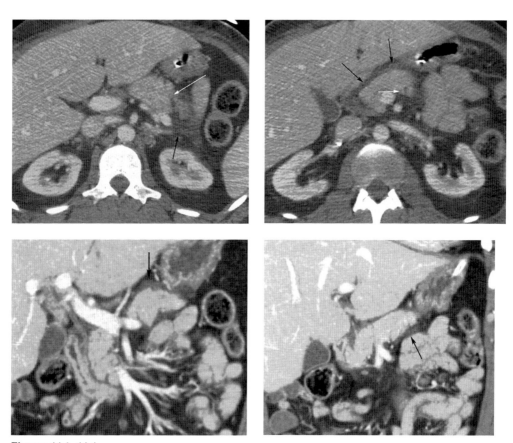

**Figures 44.1–44.4**

# Case 44  Pancreatic Injury

## Findings

### CT

▸ May be normal within the first 12 hours after injury
▸ Pancreatic enlargement, peripancreatic edema or hematoma (black arrows), with or without fluid between pancreas and splenic vein
▸ Diffuse or localized hypoattenuating area with preserved enhancement suggests contusion
▸ Hematoma appears as heterogeneous or hyperattenuating lesion
▸ Lacerations demonstrate linear low-attenuation lesions that can be difficult to see (white arrows)
▸ Ductal disruption may be identified

### MRI

▸ T1WI: Variable signal intensity
▸ T2WI: Peripancreatic fluid or pseudocyst
▸ Contrast-enhanced T1WI: Nonenhancing or hypoenhancing areas caused by contusion, laceration, fluid collection, or necrosis.
▸ MRCP may demonstrate duct compromise

## Differential Diagnosis

▸ Pancreatitis
▸ Duodenal injury or rupture
▸ "Shock" pancreas

## Teaching Points

▸ CT is the preferred initial examination
  ▪ MRCP useful for diagnosing duct injury, which is important for guiding management
▸ Commonly associated with other organ injuries (80%) or the duodenum
▸ More common with penetrating injury than blunt trauma
▸ Grading
  ▪ I: Minor hematoma or laceration without duct injury
  ▪ II: Major contusion or laceration without duct injury
  ▪ III: Distal transection or parenchymal injury with duct injury
  ▪ IV: Proximal transection or parenchymal injury involving the ampulla or bile duct
  ▪ V: Massive disruption of the pancreatic head
▸ Complications are common, occurring in 30%–60% of cases
  ▪ Postraumatic pancreatitis
  ▪ Pseudocysts
  ▪ Pancreatic duct fistulas
  ▪ Abscess

## Management

▸ Conservative management for low -grade injuries with intact duct (Grade I/II)
▸ Higher-grade injuries with ductal disruption usually require surgical management

## History

▶ 18-year-old man status post motorcycle accident.

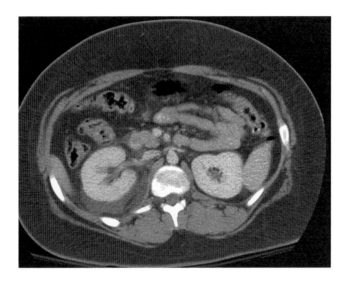

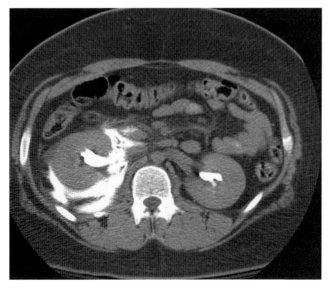

**Figures 45.1–45.2**

# Case 45 Urinoma

## Findings

### CT

► Noncontrast images show simple fluid density collection.
► Delayed images show increasing density as excreted contrast gathers in the collection.
► Located adjacent to affected kidney and/or along the course of urinary tract in the retroperitoneum and pelvis.

### Ultrasound

► Fluid collection in the perirenal space, pelvis, or retroperitoneum along the course of urinary tract.
► Intermittent signal on color Doppler from turbulence in the urinoma caused by urine flow.

## Differential Diagnosis

► Lymphocele
► Abscess
► Hematoma

## Teaching Points

► Encapsulated collection of urine caused by injury to the intrarenal or extrarenal collecting system. Most commonly located in the perirenal space.
► Etiology
  ▪ Blunt or penetrating trauma results in collecting system, ureteral, or urinary bladder injury.
  ▪ Iatrogenic causes.
  ▪ For perirenal urinomas, trauma is a more common cause. Periureteral urinomas are more commonly iatrogenic.
► Presentation: Pain, fever, hydronephrosis, and electrolyte imbalances if found late.
► Urinoma in the context of renal parenchymal injury is highly suggestive of collecting system injury (grade IV renal injury).

## Management

► Small urinomas are usually managed conservatively and usually resolve spontaneously.
► Percutaneous drainage may be considered for larger or infected urinomas.
► Nephrostomy catheters, ureteral stents, or nephroureteral catheters may also be placed to divert urine flow.

## Further Readings

Titton RL, Gervais DA, Hahn PF, Harisinghani MG, Arellano RS, Mueller PR. Urine leaks and urinomas: diagnosis and imaging–guided intervention. *RadioGraphics*. 2003;23(5):1133–1147.
Testa AC, Gaurilcikas A, Licameli A, Di Stasi C, Lorusso D, Scambia G, et al. Sonographic imaging of urinoma. *Ultrasound Obstet Gynecol*. 2009;33(4):490–491.

## History

► 45-year-old male status post motor vehicle collision.

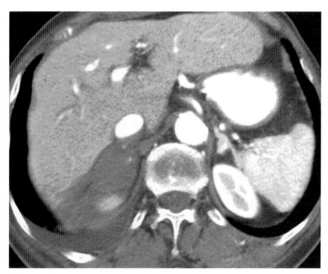

**Figure 46.1**

# Case 46  Adrenal Injury

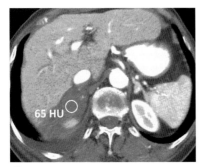

**Figure 46.2**

## Findings

### CT

▶ Hyperdense nonenhancing hematoma (50-80 HU); chronically, this will gradually decrease in size and density, and may eventually form calcifications

▶ Asymmetric round or distorted enlargement of the adrenal gland

▶ Periadrenal fat stranding or frank hemorrhage, possibly with retroperitoneal extension

▶ Other traumatic findings (i.e., fractures, pneumothorax, laceration/contusion of other solid organs)

### Ultrasound

▶ Avascular hyperechoic or hypoechoic mass; over time this will decrease in size and echogenicity, chronically becoming anechoic, possibly with shadowing calcifications

## Differential Diagnosis

▶ Adrenal hemorrhage from nontraumatic causes: Hemorrhagic adrenal mass, adrenal vein ligation/thrombosis during liver transplantation
  ▪ Bilateral adrenal hemorrhages more likely to occur from systemic etiologies, such as in the setting of anticoagulation or in situations of high stress (i.e., sepsis [Waterhouse-Friderichsen syndrome], burns, or hypotension)

▶ Adrenal hyperplasia

▶ Adrenal adenoma or myelolipoma

▶ Pheochromocytoma, adrenal carcinoma, metastasis, or lymphoma

## Teaching Points

▶ Blunt force trauma is the most common etiology

▶ Typically unilateral, right much more common than left

▶ When bilateral, it can result in a catastrophic crisis of adrenal insufficiency
  ▪ In the setting of minimal trauma with bilateral adrenal hemorrhage, a search of underlying coagulopathy is warranted

▶ If the mass does not decrease in size or resolve on follow-up CT, it may represent a disorder other than trauma and should be further evaluated as deemed clinically appropriate

## Management

▶ Therapeutic interventions for associated injuries that commonly accompany adrenal trauma

▶ Replacement steroid therapy in the setting of bilateral adrenal injury and subsequent crisis of adrenal insufficiency

▶ Adrenalectomy is typically not necessary, except in the setting where an underlying adrenal tumor is present

### Further Readings

Blake MA, Cronin CG, Boland GW. Adrenal imaging. *AJR Am J Roentgenol.* 2010 Jun;194(6):1450–60.
Mayo-Smith WW, Boland GW, Noto RB, Lee MJ. State-of-the-art adrenal imaging. *RadioGraphics.* 2001;21(4):995–1012.

## History

▶ 78-year-old male status post bladder transurethral resection of the prostate.

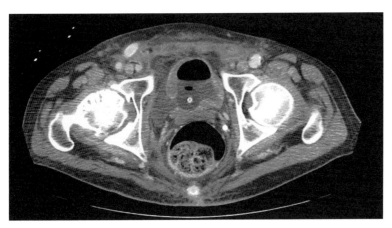

**Figure 47.1**

# Case 47  Extraperitoneal Bladder Rupture

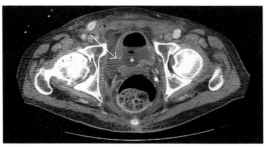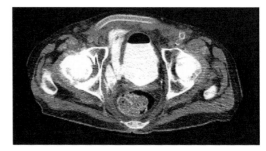

**Figures 47.2–47.3**

## Findings

▶ CT cystography demonstrates contrast extravasation into perivesical region (Figure 47.1).

▶ May see defect in the bladder wall (Figure 47.2).

▶ Complex extraperitoneal bladder rupture will also demonstrate extravasation into other perineal spaces and along the fascial planes of the abdominal wall and the thighs (Figure 47.3).

## Differential Diagnosis

▶ Intraperitoneal bladder rupture or combined extraperitoneal and intraperitoneal bladder rupture.

▶ Interstitial bladder injury where a tearing of the luminal layers of the bladder wall with an intact serosa can lead to contrast with the wall.

## Teaching Points

▶ Extraperitoneal rupture is the most common type of bladder injury.

▶ Mechanisms of injury
  ▪ Penetrating trauma
  ▪ Blunt trauma associated with pelvic fractures
  ▪ Iatrogenic (biopsy or TURP)

▶ CT cystography is absolutely indicated in the context of both gross hematuria and pelvic fractures. Less strongly indicated in patients with either gross hematuria or pelvic fracture.

▶ Grading system
  ▪ Type 1: Bladder contusion
  ▪ Type 2: Intraperitoneal rupture
  ▪ Type 3: Interstitial injury
  ▪ Type 4: Extraperitoneal rupture
  ▪ 4A: Simple extraperitoneal rupture (perivesical space)
  ▪ 4B: Complex extraperitoneal rupture (extending to scrotum, perineum, thigh)

▶ Type 5: Combined intraperitoneal and extraperitoneal rupture
  ▪ Cannot adequately assess an underdistended bladder: 300 mL of contrast filling is needed to exclude rupture.

## Management

▶ Typically, conservative treatment for extraperitoneal rupture with large-bore transurethral or suprapubic catheter.

## Further Readings

Vaccaro JP, Brody JM. CT cystography in the evaluation of major bladder trauma. *RadioGraphics*. 2000;20(5):1373–1381.
Corriere JN, Sandler CM. Diagnosis and management of bladder injuries. *Urol Clin North Am*. 2006;33(1):67–71–vi.

## History

▸ 21-year-old male with abdominal pain and hematuria following an MVA.

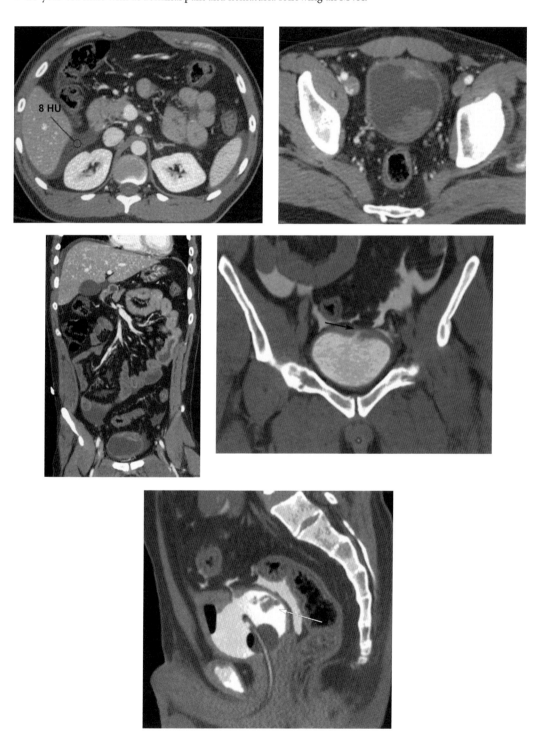

**Figures 48.1–48.5**

# Case 48  Intraperitoneal Bladder Rupture

## Findings

### Ultrasound

▶ Free intraperitoneal fluid

▶ May bladder wall irregularity/discontinuity (black arrow) or intraluminal hemorrhage (white arrow).

### Conventional Cystography

▶ Contrast extravasation into the peritoneal cavity

### CT

▶ Low-attenuation fluid in the peritoneal cavity (HU measurement)

### CT Cystography

## Differential Diagnosis

▶ Differentials for intraperitoneal fluid associated with trauma
  ▪ Simple fluid (<20 HU)
  ▪ Ascites
  ▪ Bile
  ▪ Urine
  ▪ Intermediate density (20-40 HU)
  ▪ Bowel contents (small bowel injury)
  ▪ Old blood
  ▪ High density (>40 HU)
  ▪ Blood
  ▪ Opacified bowel contents or urine

## Teaching Points

▶ Etiology
  ▪ Blunt trauma (most common): Seat belt or steering wheel injury
  ▪ Penetrating injury: Gunshot or knife wounds
  ▪ Iatrogenic injury
▶ Location of extravasation depends on site of injury. Superior rupture causes extravasation into intraperitoneal space. This is usually a result of direct pressure applied against a distended bladder.
▶ CT cystography: Bladder must be adequately distended with minimum of 300 mL diluted contrast for adults. For children, estimated filling for cystography is based on the formula: bladder capacity = 60 mL + (30 mL × age in years)
▶ Grading system
  ▪ Type 1: Bladder contusion
  ▪ Type 2: Intraperitoneal rupture
  ▪ Type 3: Interstitial injury
  ▪ Type 4: Extraperitoneal rupture (4A simple, and 4B complex)
  ▪ Type 5: Combined intraperitoneal and extraperitoneal rupture

## Management

▶ Intraperitoneal and combined intraperitoneal and extraperitoneal ruptures usually require primary surgical repair.

## History

▸ None

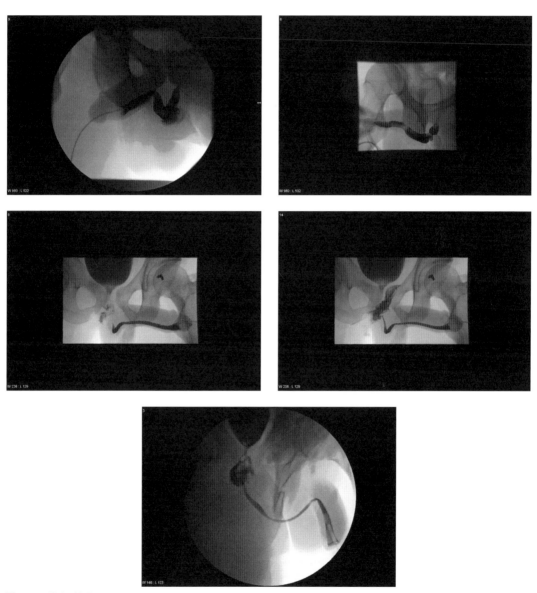

**Figures 49.1–49.5**

# Case 49  Urethral Injury

## Findings

### Retrograde Urethrography (imaging test of choice)

- Discontinuity or irregularity of the urethra
- Extravasation of contrast from the urethra
  - Partial rupture: Contrast is seen within the urethra proximal to defect
  - Complete rupture: No contrast is seen within urethra proximal to defect
- In posterior urethral injury
  - If the urogenital diaphragm remains intact, contrast is only be seen in the pelvis
  - If the urogenital diaphragm is disrupted, contrast is seen in the pelvis and the perineum

### Intravenous Urethrography

- Extravasation of contrast in voiding phase
  - Adjacent to bulbous urethra: Anterior urethral injury
  - Around the bladder base/prostate: Posterior urethral injury

### CT

- Perineal or periurethral stranding in a patient with pelvic trauma
- Ischiocavernous hematoma

## Teaching Points

- Urethral injury is seen in as many as 25% of men with pelvic fractures
- Location
  - Two-thirds involve the posterior urethra
    - Associated with pelvic fracture related to MVC or fall from height
    - Typically involves the membranous urethra
  - One-third involve the anterior urethra
    - Straddling-type injury
    - Typically involve the immobile bulbous urethra, which is crushed against an inferior pubic ramus
  - Female urethral injury is rare given short urethral length
- Classification
  - Goldman System (most widely accepted): Based on the anatomic location of the injury
  - Type 1: Urethra stretch without rupture
  - Type 2: Partial or complete rupture of the membranous urethra above the level of the urogenital diaphragm
  - Type 3: Partial or complete rupture of the membranous urethra with disruption of the urogenital diaphragm
  - Type 4: Bladder neck injury with extension into the urethra
  - Type 5: Isolated anterior urethral injury
- Stricture is a common late complication of anterior urethral injury, seen in as many at two-thirds of patients

## Management

- Partial rupture: Placement of a urethral catheter for 2–3 weeks to allow urethral healing; follow-up urethography to confirm healing
- Complete rupture: Surgical repair
  - Surgical repair 3–6 months to allow pelvic hematoma to resolve
  - Suprapubic catheter is placed to divert urine

## History

▸ Motorcycle accident.

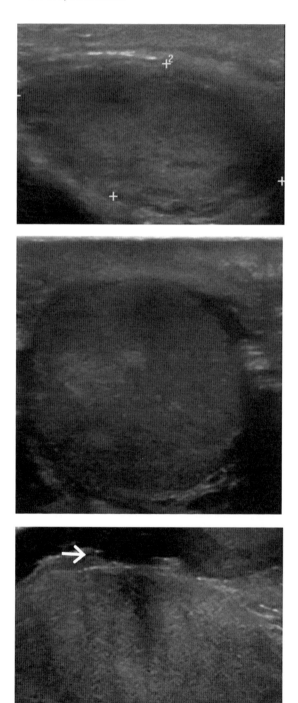

**Figures 50.1–50.3**

# Case 50  Scrotal/Testicular Injury

### Findings

▸ Testicular contour is ill-defined on ultrasound (Figures 50.1 and 50.2).
▸ Heterogeneous echotexture of the testicular parenchyma (Figures 50.1 and 50.2).
▸ Interruption of the tunica may be directly visualized (Figure 50.3).
▸ May also see abnormal or absent vascularity within a portion of the testis.
▸ Linear hypoechoic band without vascularity can indicate testicular fracture, a rarer injury.
▸ Hematoma may be seen within the testis; within the tunica vaginalis (hematocele); within the scrotal wall; or within the spermatic cord.

### Teaching Points

▸ Testicular rupture is protrusion of the seminiferous tubules through a tear in the tunica albuginea (arrow).
  ▪ Most occur from blunt trauma
  ▪ Blunt trauma usually requires higher specificity of clinical and imaging findings for surgical exploration than penetrating trauma
  ▪ Ultrasound evaluation is particularly useful in the setting of blunt trauma
▸ Various testicular injuries have overlapping sonographic features, and a heterogeneous appearance can reflect testicular hematoma and/or contusion (injured, devitalized tissue), with or without the presence of rupture.
  ▪ Rupture should, therefore, not be diagnosed based on heterogeneity alone
  ▪ Hypoechoic avascular linear tissue defects reflect shear injury (testicular fracture) and may be seen concurrently with other injuries
▸ The combined findings of heterogeneous echotexture and an ill-defined contour of the testicle have high sensitivity and specificity for rupture.
  ▪ Adjacent hematoma can simulate a testicular contour abnormality, and so the contour abnormality is considered an indirect sign of rupture
  ▪ Heterogeneity concurrent with tissue interruption at surface of the testicle (direct observation of tunica albuginea tear) is highly specific for rupture, but the latter finding is often difficult to make
▸ Testicular hematoma requires follow-up imaging to resolution.
  ▪ Partly, this is to evaluate for the development of necrosis and infection of the hematoma.
  ▪ In addition, testicular tumors can present as pain related to minor trauma and simulate the appearance of hematoma on ultrasound.
▸ Traumatic testicular torsion has a similar ultrasound appearance to nontraumatic torsion.

### Management

▸ Most testicular ruptures can be surgically repaired when detected promptly.
▸ Extensive rupture requires orchiectomy.
▸ Intratesticular hematomas require imaging follow-up.

**History**

► Trauma

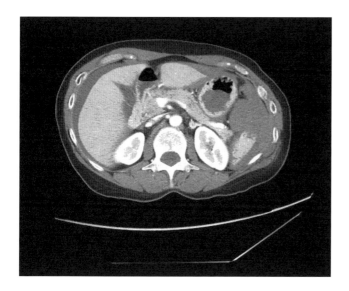

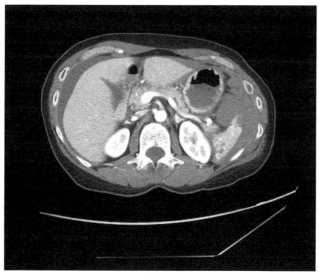

**Figures 51.1–51.2**

# Case 51  Hemoperitoneum

**Findings**

**US**

- ▶ Hypoechoic free fluid in the peritoneal cavity
- ▶ May see some complexity in this fluid depending on age
- ▶ Must differentiate bowel contents and physiologic fluid

**CT**

- ▶ Hyperdense fluid within the peritoneal cavity typically measuring between 30 and 60 HU
- ▶ May see "sentinel clot," where highest-density material gathers around an injured organ
- ▶ May see focal area with density similar to adjacent vessel, suggestive of active extravasation
- ▶ Triangular collections of blood in mesenteric reflections usually indicate mesenteric source of bleeding

**Differential Diagnosis**

- ▶ Intraperitoneal free fluid
  - ▪ Simple ascites
  - ▪ Bile, secondary to biliary injury
  - ▪ Urine, secondary to urinary tract injury
  - ▪ Chyle, secondary to lymphatic injury
  - ▪ Intestinal contents, related to bowel injury
- ▶ High-attenuation ascites on CT
  - ▪ Infection especially tuberculosis
  - ▪ Malignancy, such as ovarian/appendiceal tumor (pseudomyxoma)
  - ▪ Ascitic fluid on a background of severe fatty liver
- ▶ Mimics of hemoperitoneum on US
  - ▪ Fluid-filled bowel loops
  - ▪ Perinephric fat

**Teaching Points**

- ▶ Etiologies of hemoperitoneum
  - ▪ Trauma
  - ▪ Gynecologic sources: Ruptured ovarian cyst, ruptured ectopic pregnancy, ovarian torsion
  - ▪ Spontaneous hemorrhage associated with anticoagulation therapy
  - ▪ Iatrogenic, following surgery or invasive procedure
  - ▪ Highly vascular neoplasms
- ▶ Ruptured aortic or visceral artery aneurysms
- ▶ Attenuation values at CT help differentiate blood products from other sources of intraperitoneal fluid
  - ▪ Clotted blood measures 45-70 HU
  - ▪ Unclotted intraperitoneal blood usually measures 30-45 HU
  - ▪ May measure <30 HU in patients with decreased serum hematocrit level
  - ▪ Exact attenuation of blood depends on age, extent, and location of hemorrhage
- ▶ Highest attenuation hematoma or "sentinel clot" is closest to site of bleeding and may be used to identify source of bleeding
- ▶ Spleen and liver injuries are the most common solid organ injuries to result in hemoperitoneum
- ▶ Duodenum and proximal jejunum are most common sites of bowel injury giving rise to hemoperitoneum

**Management**

- ▶ Close monitoring of vital signs for evidence of hemodynamic instability
- ▶ Active extravasation and/or hemodynamic instability may indicate need for emergent surgical or endovascular treatment
- ▶ Definitive treatment through correction of underlying pathology (e.g., pseudoaneurysm coiling, splenectomy)

► Trauma

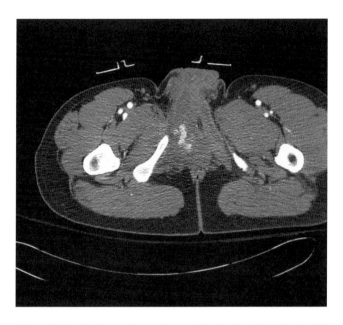

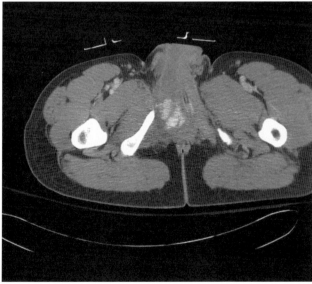

**Figures 52.1–52.2**

# Case 52   Active Extravasation

## Findings

▸ Focal area of hyperattenuation within a hematoma on initial postcontrast images
▸ On delayed images (typically at 5 minutes), the area of hyperattenuation enlarges and changes in shape and attenuation
▸ Can be found associated with solid organ injuries, muscular injuries, or direct vascular injuries

## Differential Diagnosis

▸ Pseudoaneurysm and arteriovenous fistula
▸ Opacified urine from injured renal collecting system
▸ Radiopaque foreign body or bone fragment
▸ Enteric contrast leakage from bowel injury

## Teaching Points

▸ Important indicator of morbidity and mortality in trauma patients
▸ Typically associated with active hemorrhage
▸ Localization of source of bleeding important for determining appropriate course of management
▸ Can be seen from various abdominal structures including liver, adrenal glands, kidneys, pancreas, spleen, mesentery, and soft tissues
▸ Dual-phase CT protocol with 5-minute delayed images key for differentiation from pseudoaneurysm
  ▪ Active extravasation enlarges, changes in shape, and remains hyperdense
  ▪ Pseudoaneurysm does not change in shape or size and washes out with the vascular pool
▸ Adjacent vascular structures should be evaluated for dissection, pseudoaneurysm, and lack of enhancement (caused by spasm and/or occlusion)

## Management

▸ Expectant/supportive management may be used for minor injuries, especially intramuscular or subcutaneous soft tissue injuries.
▸ Significant injuries, such as in patients with multiple injuries, or solid organ injuries, such as the spleen, may require endovascular or open surgical management.
▸ Interventions may range from intravenous fluid and transfusions of blood products to endovascular embolization, surgical ligation, or resection of injured organ.

### Further Readings

Murakami AM, Anderson SW, Soto JA, Kertesz JL, Ozonoff A, Rhea JT. Active extravasation of the abdomen and pelvis in trauma using 64MDCT. *Emerg Radiol.* 2009;16(5):375–382.
Hamilton JD, Kumaravel M, Censullo ML, Cohen AM, Kievlan DS, West OC. Multidetector CT evaluation of active extravasation in blunt abdominal and pelvic trauma patients. *RadioGraphics.* 2008;28(6):1603–1616.

## History

▸ 34-year-old man posttrauma, worsening abdominal pain.

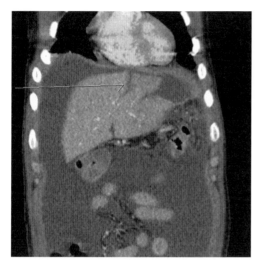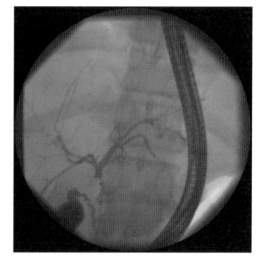

**Figures 53.1–53.2**

# Case 53  Posttraumatic bile duct leak

## Findings

- ▶ Abdominal CT with IV contrast: Jagged curvilinear hypodensities (arrow) through the left and right lobes of the liver compatible with laceration. Low-attenuation fluid around the liver and spleen and fluid in contiguity with the left lobe laceration.
- ▶ ERCP: Occlusion cholangiogram demonstrates contrast leakage from left sided biliary radicals

## Differential Diagnosis

- ▶ Simple ascites
- ▶ Hemoperitoneum from laceration of portal veins, hepatic arteries, or hepatic veins
- ▶ Peritoneal carcinomatosis and infiltrative liver metastases

## Teaching Points

- ▶ Presence of free fluid adjacent to the liver in a posttraumatic patient should raise concern for parenchymal laceration and underlying vascular or biliary injury.
- ▶ Biliary complications as a result of bile leakage caused by injury to the bile duct system include biloma, biliary fistula, bilemia, and bile peritonitis.
- ▶ At CT, progressive enlargement of a well-circumscribed, hypodense intraparenchymal or perihepatic collection after trauma strongly suggests the diagnosis of a biloma.
- ▶ Further evaluation with ERCP may be helpful to exclude biliary injury.
- ▶ Sulfur-colloid scintigraphy, or MRI with Eovist (intravenous contrast agent excreted by both the kidneys and biliary system), with delayed imaging can serve as noninvasive ways of identifying a bile duct leak.

## Management

- ▶ Percutaneous drainage, in combination with endoscopic sphinchterotomy and/or biliary stenting, can be a good initial treatment in posttraumatic bile duct injury.
- ▶ Surgical management may be needed in more complex cases.

## Further Readings

Yoon W, Jeong YY, Kim JK, Seo JJ, Lim HS, Shin SS, et al. CT in blunt liver trauma. *RadioGraphics*. 2005;25:87–104.
Haney PJ, Whitley NO, Brotman S, Cunat JS, Whitley J. Liver injury and complications in the postoperative trauma patient: CT evaluation. *AJR Am J Roentgenol*. 1982;139(2):271–275.

## History

▸ MVA

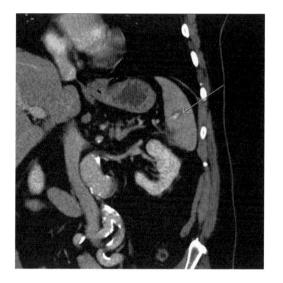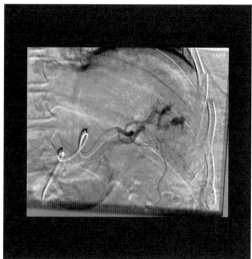

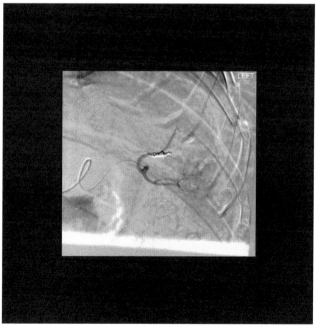

**Figures 54.1–54.3**

# Case 54  Splenic Injury/Laceration

## Findings

### CT

▶ Coronal images with IV contrast demonstrating a splenic laceration with active extravasation (arrow)

### Arterial Angiogram

▶ Pre-embolization and postembolization demonstrating an active bleeding/pseudoaneurysm in the spleen

## Teaching Points

▶ The spleen is the most commonly injured organ after blunt trauma to the abdomen.
▶ The American Association for the Surgery of Trauma (AAST) splenic injury grading system:
  ▪ Grade I
    ▪ Subcapsular hematoma <10% surface area
    ▪ Capsular laceration <1 cm depth
  ▪ Grade II
    ▪ Subcapsular hematoma 10%–50% surface area
    ▪ Intraparenchymal hematoma <5 cm
    ▪ Laceration 1–3 cm depth not involving trabecular vessels
  ▪ Grade III
    ▪ Subcapsular hematoma >50% of surface area or expanding
    ▪ Intraparenchymal hematoma >5 cm/expanding
    ▪ Laceration >3 cm depth or involving trabecular vessels
    ▪ Ruptured subcapsular or parenchymal hematoma
  ▪ Grade IV
    ▪ Laceration involving segmental/hilar vessels with major devascularization (>25% of spleen)
  ▪ Grade V
    ▪ Shattered spleen
    ▪ Hilar vascular injury with devascularized spleen
▶ The focused assessment with sonography in trauma (FAST) examination is more useful in hemodynamically unstable patients; however, a negative examination does not exclude splenic injury.
▶ The diagnostic peritoneal lavage (DPL) is largely replaced by the FAST in most major trauma centers.
▶ Pitfalls in diagnosis of splenic injury
  ▪ Normal lobulation/cleft mimics tear
  ▪ Adjacent nonopacified bowel loop (jejunum) may look like laceration
  ▪ Too early acquisition of scan after bolus spleen can appear inhomogeneous (differential enhancement of red and white pulp)
  ▪ Previous infarct
  ▪ Perisplenic fluid from ascites or lavage

## Management

▶ Hemodynamically unstable: patient with a positive FAST scan or DPA/DPL requires emergent abdominal exploration.
▶ Hemodynamically stable: patients with low-grade (I–III) blunt or penetrating splenic injuries without any evidence for other intra-abdominal injuries, active contrast extravasation, may be initially observed safely.
▶ The use of nonsurgical management as the first-line therapeutic step in adults has been advocated by The Eastern Association for the Surgery of Trauma Practice Management Guidelines Working Group.
▶ Surgery is usually performed in patients who have traumatic injuries to the spleen and unstable hemodynamics.
▶ The splenic arterial embolization is mostly used with evidence of arterial injury on CT scans. With nonoperative management, splenic function is preserved, and the lifelong risk of postsplenectomy sepsis, surgery complications, hospitalization periods, and costs are lower.

**History**

▶ Trauma

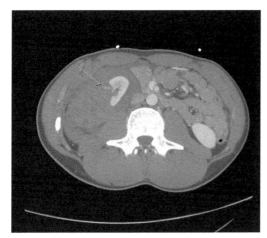 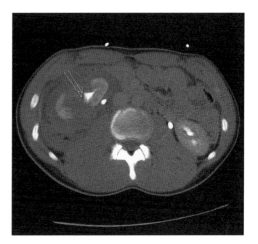

**Figures 55.1–55.2**

# Case 55  Renal Laceration with Hematoma, Vascular Extravasation, and Urine Extravasation

## Findings

▶ Axial CT with contrast demonstrating right kidney injury with contrast extravasation (arrow). There is an extensive hematoma surrounding the kidney.

▶ Axial CT, with delayed imaging demonstrating urine leak (double arrows).

## Teaching Points

▶ Arterial-phase CT is useful to help delineate renal arterial injury, but nephrographic and urinary phase imaging may also be necessary to fully delineate renal injuries.

▶ Delayed CT images are important to check for urine leak, which is typically treated with placement of ureteral stent. Delayed CT is also useful to separate extravasated urine (which accumulates) from extravasated arterial contrast material, which dilutes after the bolus is stopped.

▶ Lacerations connecting the cortical surfaces through the hilum are termed fractures. Multiple separated renal fragments, which may or may not be perfused, are termed shattered.

▶ AAST grading system (1)
  ▪ Grade I
    ▪ Contusion; or
    ▪ Nonexpanding subcapsular hematoma
  ▪ Grade II
    ▪ Nonexpanding perirenal hematoma; or
    ▪ Laceration <1 cm deep into the renal cortex
  ▪ Grade III
    ▪ Laceration >1 cm but not extending to the collecting system
  ▪ Grade IV
    ▪ Laceration extending to the collecting system; or
    ▪ Main renal artery/vein injury
  ▪ Grade V
    ▪ Shattered kidney; or
    ▪ Renal hilum avulsion

▶ Chronic subcapsular hematoma can lead to compression necrosis of parenchyma (the Page kidney phenomenon), a rare cause of secondary hypertension and renal failure.

## Management

▶ Patients with hematuria of <35 red blood cells per high-power field, with no history of hypotension, and with no pelvic fracture can usually forego imaging of the urinary tract.

▶ Parenchymal contusions and minor superficial lacerations do not necessitate surgery in 95% of cases (2).

▶ Major renal lacerations with urine leak in stable patients may be treated nonsurgically, with observation, serial imaging, and placement of a stent in the ureter (3).

▶ Injuries with persistent large urine leak, ureteropelvic junction avulsion, enlarging central and subcapsular hematoma, or extensively devitalized parenchyma (particularly in an immunocompromised patient) need surgical intervention.

# Section 5    Upper Extremity

## History

► Trauma to right shoulder region.

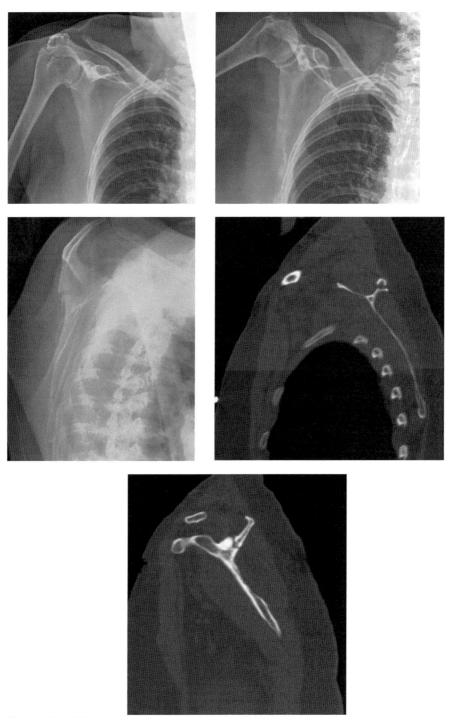

**Figures 56.1–56.5**

# Case 56  Scapular Fracture

## Findings

### Radiography

▶ On the AP radiograph view of right shoulder it is difficult to appreciate the cortical discontinuity involving the spine of the scapula. Additional scapular views demonstrate this fracture to better advantage.

▶ This is also evident on the scapular Y-view.

▶ There is normal glenohumeral alignment and no additional fracture.

### CT

▶ The fracture of the spine of the scapula is confirmed on CT. It extended into the suprascapular notch but not to the glenoid articular surface.

## Teaching Points

▶ Fractures of the scapula are relatively rare injuries; they represent 3%–5% of all fractures involving the shoulder girdle and 1% of fractures overall.

▶ Direct trauma to the lateral or posterosuperior aspect of the forequarter is the most common mechanism of injury. Ninety percent of patients who sustain scapular fractures have other associated injuries. Because attention is often directed initially toward these other injuries, fractures of the scapula are often initially overlooked.

▶ Fractures that involve the glenoid neck and scapular body are the most common

▶ There is a high incidence of pneumothorax, occurring in half of patients. Most are delayed in onset, occurring 1–3 days after the injury. Some authors advocate a follow-up chest radiograph.

## Management

▶ If nonoperative treatment is chosen, the shoulder is immobilized for comfort. Passive exercises are initiated early and active-assisted range of motion exercises are begun once there is evidence of union.

▶ The decision to proceed to surgical treatment is primarily based on the degree of displacement.

▶ If surgery is considered, it is usually performed through a posterior approach. Screw fixation alone is not usually sufficient because of the thin quality of the scapular bone. Plate fixation with horizontally or obliquely oriented plates with multiple screws is therefore usually necessary to obtain stability.

## Further Readings

Lapner PC, Uhthoff HK, Papp S. Scapula fractures. *Orthop Clin North Am*. 2008;39(4):459–474, vi. PMID: 18803976
Cole PA, Gauger EM, Schroder LK. Management of scapular fractures. *J Am Acad Orthop Surg*. 2012;20(3):130–141. PMID: 2238228

## History

▶ 48-year-old man in motor vehicle accident.

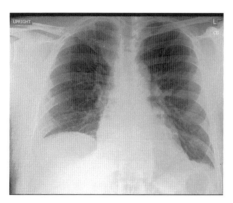

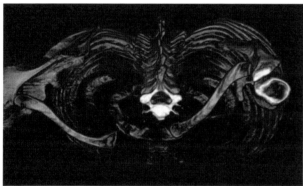

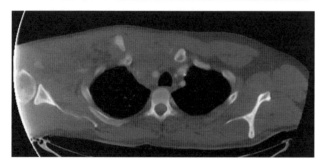

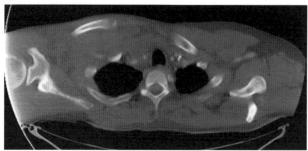

**Figures 57.1–57.4**

# Case 57  Sternoclavicular Dislocation

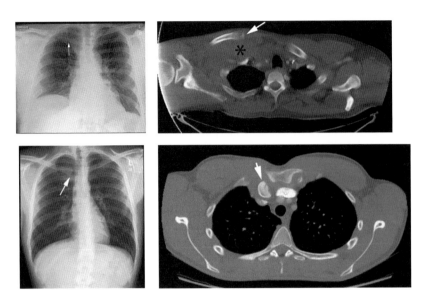

**Figures 57.5–57.8**

## Findings

► Radiographic diagnosis is often difficult because of superimposition of structures and the oblique orientation of the joint. Abnormal position or asymmetry of the medial clavicles is the key radiographic finding (arrows).

► CT is the preferred imaging modality. It depicts alignment at the sternoclavicular joint and direction of dislocation of the medial clavicular head, either anterior or posterior (arrows). The great vessels, trachea, esophagus, and associated hematoma (asterisk) are also well evaluated.

## Differential Diagnosis

► Spontaneous atraumatic anterior sternoclavicular dislocation: Uncommon condition, primarily in teenagers and young adults, caused by ligamentous laxity. Dislocation occurs with overhead positioning of the arm.

► Medial clavicular epiphyseal fracture: Salter-Harris type I fracture of the medial end of the clavicle may mimic sternoclavicular dislocation. The medial clavicular epiphysis is the last epiphysis to ossify (at ~19 years) and close (at 23–25 years).

## Teaching Points

► Sternoclavicular dislocation is rare.

► The medial clavicle may dislocate anteriorly (presternal) or posteriorly (retrosternal) relative to the sternum.

► Anterior dislocation, which is more common, is caused by posteriorly directed trauma to the shoulder, which levers the medial clavicle anteriorly.

► Posterior dislocation is usually caused by indirect trauma where a force applied to the posterolateral shoulder causes anterior displacement of the lateral clavicle and levering of the medial clavicle posteriorly. Alternatively, posterior dislocation may result from high-energy direct trauma to the medial clavicle where it may be associated with other chest injuries, including pulmonary contusion and rib fractures.

► Posterior dislocation of the medial clavicle may result in significant morbidity and mortality, which may present with dyspnea, dysphagia, brachial plexopathy, or venous congestion in the neck.

## Management

► Anterior dislocation is initially managed with closed reduction, which although typically leaves residual deformity, yields good functional outcomes without surgical risk. If this fails, arthroplasty is necessary.

► Posterior dislocation is usually initially treated with closed reduction. Open reduction is performed when closed reduction fails or when there is mediastinal involvement. The joint is usually stable postreduction.

► None

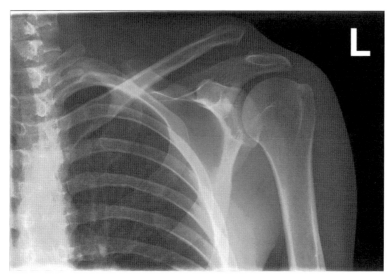

**Figure 58.1**

# Case 58  Acromioclavicular (AC) Joint Separation (Type III)

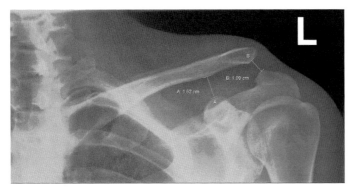

**Figure 58.2**

## Findings

▶ Injury to acromioclavicular joint supporting structures (including coracoclavicular ligaments)

### Subtypes (Rockwood classification)

▶ Type I: Acromioclavicular ligament sprain without ligamentous tear
  ▪ No imaging abnormality, no joint malalignment
▶ Type II: Acromioclavicular ligament tear
  ▪ Increased acromioclavicular distance >5–6 mm on AP view
    ▪ Normal anatomic variation: no >3 mm difference from contralateral
    ▪ May be partial tear of ligaments and require stress views with weights to diagnose
▶ Type III: Complete tear of acromioclavicular and coracoclavicular ligaments
  ▪ Superior displacement of clavicle
    ▪ Increased coracoclavicular distance >11–13 mm on AP view
    ▪ Normal anatomic variation: no >5 mm difference from contralateral
▶ Type IV: Complete tear of acromioclavicular and coracoclavicular ligaments with posterior displacement of clavicle
  ▪ Because superior displacement may be absent, AP view may appear normal; need axillary view to detect posterior displacement
▶ Type V: Complete tear of acromioclavicular and coracoclavicular ligaments and torn muscular attachments to clavicle (deltoid and trapezius) with SUPERIOR displacement of clavicle
▶ Type VI: Complete tear of acromioclavicular and coracoclavicular ligaments with INFERIOR displacement of clavicle (rare)

## Differential Diagnosis

▶ Normal anatomic variation
▶ Clavicle fracture

## Teaching Points

▶ Mechanism
  ▪ Direct blow to superior aspect of shoulder, usually from fall (most common)
  ▪ Fall on outstretched hand (less common)

## Management

▶ Treatment
  ▪ Type I: Conservative (rest, pain control, activity modification)
  ▪ Type II: Conservative (rest, pain control, activity modification)
  ▪ Type III: Mostly conservative; some opt for surgical management if vocation/avocation requires heavy lifting
  ▪ Type IV–VI: Surgical fixation

## History

▶ None

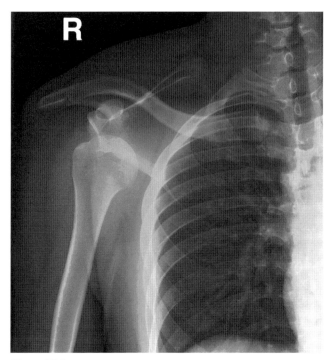

**Figure 59.1**

# Case 59  Anterior Shoulder Dislocation

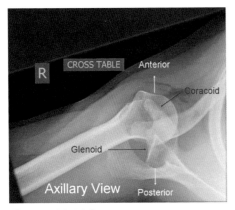
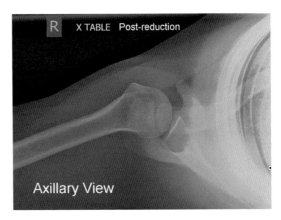

**Figures 59.2–59.3**

## Findings

▶ Humeral head displaced medial and inferior relative to glenoid fossa on AP view; humeral head lies inferior to coracoid
▶ Orthogonal view required for confirmation of anterior displacement

## Associated Findings

▶ Fracture of anterior glenoid rim (Bankart fracture) less common; anterior inferior labral injury (soft tissue Bankart lesion) common
▶ Impaction fracture of posterior lateral humeral head where it contacts the anterior inferior glenoid (Hill-Sachs lesion); up to 80% incidence with anterior dislocation
▶ Soft tissue injuries (on MRI)

## Differential Diagnosis

▶ Inferior dislocation
▶ Posterior dislocation

## Teaching Points

▶ Mechanism: Position of greatest vulnerability is abduction and external rotation
  ▪ Forced external rotation or extension while in abduction
  ▪ Direct blow to posterior shoulder (e.g., from fall)
  ▪ Fall on outstretched hand
  ▪ Common: 95% of glenohumeral dislocations

## Management

▶ CT
  ▪ More sensitive for glenoid fractures
▶ MRI
  ▪ Evaluate associated soft tissue pathology
    ▪ Labrum
    ▪ Rotator cuff
    ▪ Inferior glenohumeral ligament

## Treatment

▶ Closed reduction (+/- anesthesia)
▶ Open reduction (reserved for extreme cases with locked humeral head)
▶ Treatment of associated fractures and soft tissue injury.

## History

▶ None

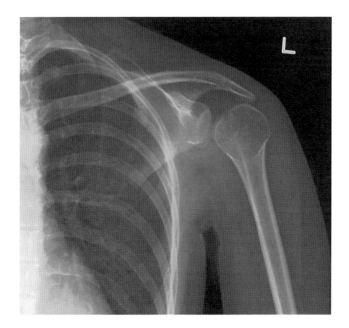

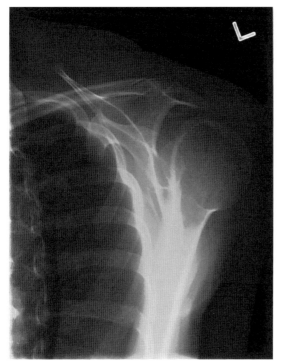

**Figures 60.1–60.2**

# Case 60   Posterior Shoulder Dislocation

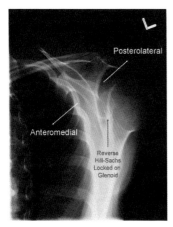

**Figure 60.3**

## Findings

▶ Humeral head dislocated posterior and lateral to glenoid fossa

## Diagnosis

▶ Lateral translocation of humeral head relative to glenoid fossa on AP view
  ▪ Overlap of glenoid and humeral head is decreased or absent
  ▪ Glenohumeral joint space >6 mm
  ▪ If dislocated far enough posterior, may appear in normal medial-lateral position
▶ Humerus fixed in internal rotation
  ▪ Humeral head appears like a "lightbulb" because of medialization of lesser tuberosity

## Associated findings

▶ Trough sign or reversed Hill-Sachs

## Differential Diagnosis

▶ Anterior dislocation
▶ Inferior dislocation

## Teaching Points
### Mechanism

▶ Seizure
▶ Electric shock
▶ Fall on outstretched hand
▶ Vulnerable position is flexion, adduction, and internal rotation
▶ Uncommon: <5% of glenohumeral dislocations

### Complications

▶ Humeral head may become locked on glenoid rim

## Management
### Treatment

▶ Closed reduction (+/- anesthesia)
▶ Open reduction (reserved for extreme cases with locked humeral head)
▶ Treatment of associated fractures and soft tissue injury

## History

▶ Trauma to right shoulder region.

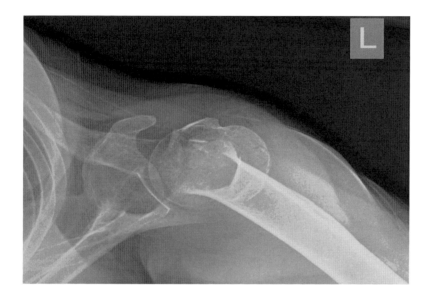

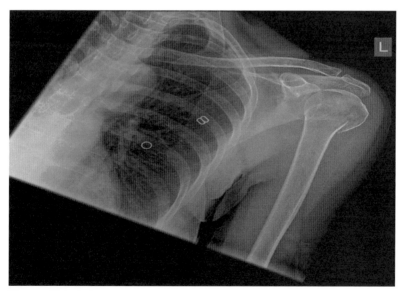

**Figures 61.1–61.2**

# Case 61  Humerus Fracture, Proximal

### Findings

▶ There is a mildly displaced fracture of the proximal humerus at the metadiaphysis.

▶ No intra-articular extension identified; no dislocation

### Differential Diagnosis

▶ None

### Teaching Points

▶ Proximal humeral fractures are common injuries accounting for 4%–5% of all fractures and are the third most common fracture in patients older than 65 years of age.

▶ Surgical neck fractures are extracapsular, usually have an adequate blood supply, and relatively low incidence of AVN; in contrast, anatomic neck fractures have a much higher incidence of AVN.

▶ In older patients they follow low-energy trauma, such as a fall on an outstretched hand from a standing height. This can lead to marked comminution caused by osteoporosis. In younger patients they are higher-energy injuries and a fracture-dislocation can occur as the capsuloligamentous structures fail before the bone.

▶ Anatomic neck fractures occur just below the articular surface. They are rare and have a poor prognosis because of loss of the blood supply to the head fragment.

▶ Surgical neck fractures occur between the level of the tuberosities and the insertion of pectoralis major. They are extracapsular and the blood supply to the head is preserved.

### Management

▶ Nonoperative treatment for stable proximal humeral fractures (stability is present when the patient can actively move extremity without pain, and limb can be moved passively with little pain and no abnormal motion between fragments).

▶ Operative management for unstable fractures, using percutaneous screws, plate, and screw constructs, or hemiarthroplasty depending on severity.

### Further Readings

Harrison JW, Howcroft DW, Warner JG, Hodgson SP. Internal fixation of proximal humeral fractures. *Acta Orthop Belg.* 2007;73(1):1–11. PMID: 17441651

Robinson CM, Amin AK, Godley KC, Murray IR, White TO. Modern perspectives of open reduction and plate fixation of proximal humerus fractures. *J Orthop Trauma.* 2011;25(10):618–629. PMID: 21904170

**History**

▸ Trauma to right elbow region

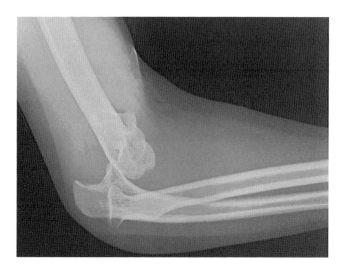

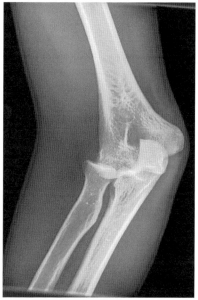

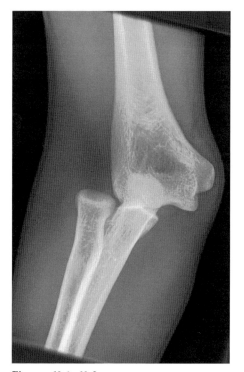

**Figures 62.1–62.3**

# Case 62   Elbow Dislocation

## Findings

### Radiography

▶ There is posterior, lateral, and proximal displacement of the radius and ulna relative to the distal humerus.

▶ No displaced fracture identified. There is some associated soft tissue swelling.

## Differential Diagnosis

▶ None

## Teaching Points

▶ The elbow is the second most commonly dislocated joint in the body behind the shoulder in the adult population.

▶ Simple dislocations represent dissociation of the ulnohumeral joint without concomitant fracture. Complex instability occurs when a fracture is associated with dislocation. Bony injuries associated with dislocation include radial head and neck fractures, coronoid fractures, and avulsion of the medial and/or lateral epicondyles.

▶ Simple elbow dislocations are classified by the direction of displacement as posterior, anterior, or divergent based on the relationship of the ulna and radius to the humerus. The most common direction of dislocation is posterior with the forearm positioned either medial or lateral to the humerus.

## Management

▶ Once a stable reduction is obtained, most simple dislocations can be managed nonoperatively with splinting or bracing, guided by the degree of instability determined during postreduction examination.

▶ Surgical management of simple elbow dislocation is indicated in elbows that remain unstable, even when placed in flexion and pronation. These elbows typically have extensive soft tissue injury involving the lateral and ulnar collateral ligaments, the common extensor and flexor-pronator muscle attachments, and the anterior capsule.

## Further Readings

Rosas HG, Lee KS. Imaging acute trauma of the elbow. *Semin Musculoskelet Radiol.* 2010;14(4):394–411. PMID: 20827621

Parsons BO, Ramsey ML. Acute elbow dislocations in athletes. *Clin Sports Med.* 2010;29(4):599–609. PMID: 20883899

Morrey BF. Current concepts in the management of complex elbow trauma. *Surgeon.* 2009;7(3):151–161. PMID: 19580179

## History

▸ Trauma to right elbow region.

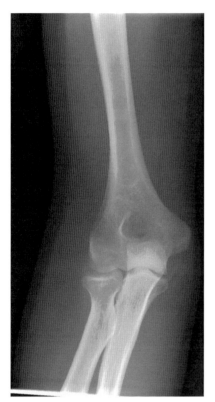 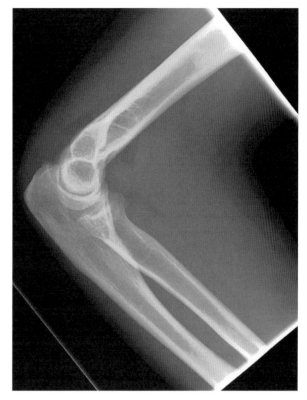

**Figures 63.1–63.2**

# Case 63   Radial Head Fracture

## Findings

### Radiography

▶ There is an impacted comminuted fracture of the lateral articular surface of the radial head (straight arrow).

▶ The lateral radiograph demonstrates a large elbow joint effusion with a "sail-sign" anteriorly (curved arrow) that represents the displaced anterior fat pad. In addition the posterior fat pad is visible consistent with a large effusion.

## Teaching Points

▶ Radial head fractures are the most common type of elbow fractures. Fractures are classified based on the degree of displacement, size of articular fragment, and degree of comminution.

▶ They are usually caused by a fall on the outstretched hand, with the elbow flexed. Axial and valgus loading shears the radial head against the capitellum.

▶ Comminuted head fractures often signify a high-energy injury, although in osteoporotic bone they can result from simple falls. Comminuted radial head fractures are the marker of a significant and extensive elbow injury that only rarely, if ever, occurs in isolation. Comminuted radial head fractures have been associated with ligamentous injuries, proximal ulnar and capitellar fractures, and forearm interosseous membrane disruption.

▶ Radiographs of both wrists should be obtained when the clinical examination reveals forearm or ulnar-sided wrist pain that is suggestive of injury to the interosseous ligament.

▶ CT with sagittal, coronal, and three-dimensional reconstructions may assist with preoperative planning and can help the surgeon predict whether a displaced radial head fracture can be treated with ORIF or whether an arthroplasty is needed.

## Management

▶ Nonoperative management is favored for undisplaced fractures.

▶ Options for the treatment of displaced fractures include nonoperative management, fragment excision, whole head excision, open reduction and internal fixation, and radial head arthroplasty.

### Further Readings

Rosenblatt Y, Athwal GS, Faber KJ. Current recommendations for the treatment of radial head fractures. *Orthop Clin North Am.* 2008;39(2):173–185. PMID: 1837480

Ring D. Radial head fracture: open reduction-internal fixation or prosthetic replacement. *J Shoulder Elbow Surg.* 2011;20(Suppl 2):S107–S112. PMID: 21281915

## History

▶ 40-year-old man status post fall on an outstretched hand.

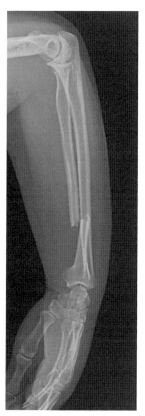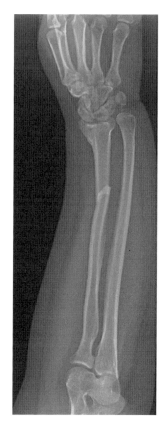

**Figures 64.1–64.2**

# Case 64  Galeazzi Fracture-Dislocation

## Findings

► Fracture of the radial shaft with dislocation of the distal radioulnar joint (DRUJ)
► Radial shaft fracture usually involves the middle to distal third
► DRUJ dislocation is usually dorsal because of shortening and rotation by the brachioradialis and rotation of the distal fragment toward the ulna by the pronator quadratus

## Differential Diagnosis

► Monteggia fracture-dislocation
► Essex-Lopresti
► Isolated radial shaft fracture

## Teaching Points

► Etiology
  ▪ Fall on an outstretched hand with a flexed elbow
  ▪ High-energy direct blow with forearm pronation
► Epidemiology: Uncommon, 3%–7% of all forearm fractures; more common in males
► Two types
  ▪ Type I: Fracture within 7.5 cm of midarticular surface of the distal radius. Greater chance of DRUJ instability, potentially requiring K wire fixation.
  ▪ Type II: Fracture >7.5 cm from the joint surface.
  ▪ The closer the radial shaft fracture to the DRUJ, the more likely the joint becomes unstable.
► CT is the best method to evaluate the DRUJ in uncertain cases

## Management

► Most adults require open reduction internal fixation.

### Further Readings

Giannoulis FS, Sotereanos DG. Galeazzi fractures and dislocations. *Hand Clin.* 2007;23:153–163.
Rettig ME, Raskin KB. Galeazzi fracture-dislocation: a new treatment-oriented classification. *J Hand Surg Am.* 2001;26(2) 228–235.

## History

▶ Trauma to wrist region.

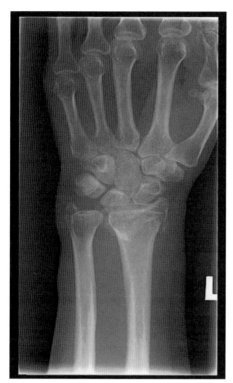 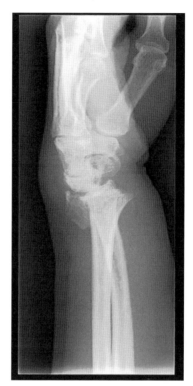

**Figures 65.1–65.2**

# Case 65   Colles Fracture

## Findings

There is an impacted comminuted intra-articular fracture of the distal radius with dorsal displacement and angulation of the distal fragment. In addition there is a fracture of the distal ulnar styloid.

## Differential Diagnosis

► Smith fracture
► Barton fracture
► Die-punch fracture

## Teaching Points

► Fractures of the distal radius are very common, with an incidence ranging between 10% and 25% of all fractures.
► The Colles fracture was first described by Abraham Colles, an Irish surgeon, in 1814 before the advent of radiography. Typically the distal radial fragment is dorsally displaced and angulated with resultant "dinner fork" deformity.
► The usual victim is a middle-aged or elderly woman who falls on the outstretched palm of her hand, force being translated upward to the glenohumeral articulation of the shoulder.
► Smith fractures occur in younger patients and are the result of high-energy trauma on the volar flexed wrist. Volar comminution and intra-articular extension are more common. A Barton fracture only involves the rim of the radius and can be volar or dorsal. Dislocation of the radiocarpal joint is the hallmark of Barton fractures.
► A die-punch fracture is a depression fracture of the lunate fossa of the distal radius. It is the result of a transverse load through the lunate.

## Management

► Anatomic reduction with stable fixation is the treatment of choice for displaced, unstable fractures of the distal part of the radius. The goals of treatment are to restore the articular surface congruency and to restore the radial height, radial inclination, and palmar tilt.
► CT is a useful radiographic adjunct and is recommended in the assessment of intraarticular distal radius fractures when the fracture pattern, the extent of comminution, or the magnitude and direction of the displacement of the fracture fragments cannot be determined with certainty on plain radiograph.
► Untreated fractures of the base of the ulnar styloid result in high rates of nonunion and have been associated with distal radioulnar joint instability. The role of internal fixation of the ulnar styloid is controversial.

**History**

▸ None

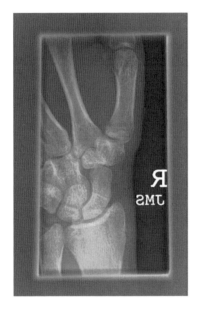

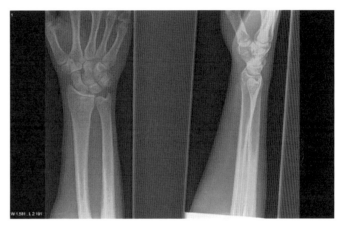

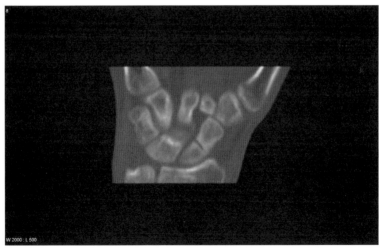

**Figures 66.1–66.3**

# Case 66   Scaphoid Fracture

## Findings

▶ Plain film: Disruption of cortex or trabecula most commonly along the middle third (waist); normal if occult fracture
▶ CT: Disruption of cortex or trabecula; better defines fracture displacement and angulation
▶ MRI: T1 hypointense fracture line; T2 hyperintense bone marrow edema; postcontrast images help determine fracture fragment viability; best to evaluate occult fractures and ligamentous injury
▶ Chronic complications
  ▪ Malunion: "humpback" deformity
  ▪ Delayed union: Incomplete union after 4 months
  ▪ Nonunion: Failure to heal after 6 months (persistent fracture line and sclerotic margins of bone)
  ▪ Osteonecrosis: Fragmentation and collapse; T1 and T2 dark bone

## Differential Diagnosis

▶ Intraosseous vascular vessel
▶ Nonunion from prior trauma
▶ Partial coalition (extremely rare)

## Teaching Points

▶ Most common carpal bone fracture and most commonly fractured at the waist.
▶ Blood supply from radial artery enters at the waist and supplies the proximal bone in a retrograde fashion. This makes the proximal fracture fragment vulnerable to osteonecrosis.

## Management

▶ Cast immobilization for stable and nondisplaced
▶ Closed reduction with percutaneous pin or screw fixation or ORIF for displaced or unstable fractures.

## Further Readings

Kaewlai R, Avery LL, Asrani AV, et al. Multidetector CT of carpal injuries: anatomy, fractures, and fracture-dislocations. *RadioGraphics.* 2008;28:1771–1784.
Cassidy C, Leonard R. Fractures and dislocations of the carpus. In: *Skeletal Trauma: Basic Science, Management, and Reconstruction.* Philadelphia, PA: Saunders/Elsevier, Vol. 1. 2009:1343–1360.
Breitenseher MJ, Metz VM, Gilula LA, et al. Radiographically occult scaphoid fractures: value of MR imaging in detection. *Radiology.* 1997;203:245–250.

Case 67

**History**
- None

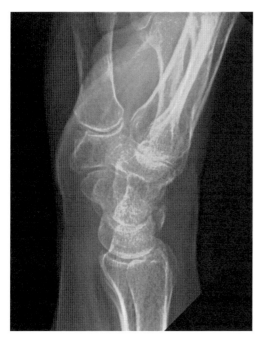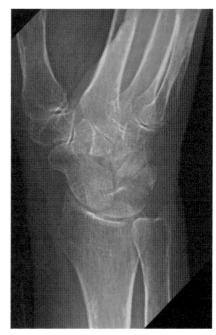

**Figures 67.1–67.2**

145

# Case 67  Triquetral Fracture: Dorsal Avulsion

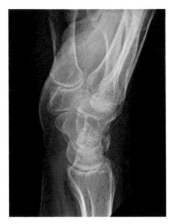

**Figure 67.3**

### Findings

▶ Avulsion fracture of the dorsal aspect of the triquetrum from traction at the insertion of the dorsal intercarpal (trapezoidal-triquetral) and radiotriquetral ligaments (arrows)

### Diagnosis

▶ Lateral radiograph of wrist
  ▪ Ossific fragment dorsal to triquetrum
▶ May also be seen on oblique view
▶ Rarely identifiable on AP view
▶ Associated findings
  ▪ Triangular fibrocartilage injury
  ▪ Lunotriquetral ligament injury

### Differential Diagnosis

▶ Acute versus chronic fracture
▶ Carpal fracture-dislocation

### Teaching Points

▶ Second most common carpal bone fracture after scaphoid fracture
▶ Three types
  ▪ Dorsal avulsion (most common; >90% of triquetral fractures)
    ▪ Often occurs in isolation
  ▪ Volar avulsion
  ▪ Triquetral body fracture (rare)
    ▪ Usually direct blow
    ▪ Associated with perilunate dislocation
▶ Mechanism: Fall on outstretched hand; hyperextension or hyperflexion of wrist with axial loading

### Management

▶ Further imaging: MRI if suspicion of associated soft tissue
▶ Treatment: Immobilization; most fractures progress to asymptomatic fibrous union

Further Reading

Goldfarb CA, Yin Y, Gilula LA, et al. Wrist fractures: what the clinician wants to know. *Radiology*. 2001;219:11–28.

Case 68

History

► None

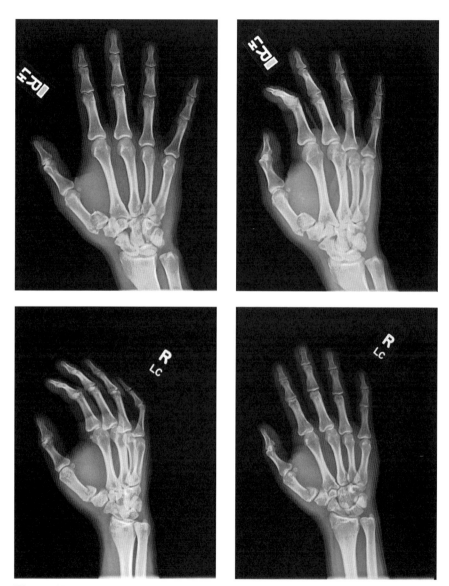

**Figures 68.1–68.4**

147

# Case 68  First Metacarpal Fracture

### Findings

#### Bennett

▶ Oblique two-part fracture at base of first metacarpal extending into the carpometacarpal joint.

  ▪ Causes dorsolateral dislocation of the main metacarpal shaft with a smaller triangular volar lip fragment remaining attached to the trapezium by the anterior oblique ligament

#### Rolando

▶ Comminuted fracture at base of first metacarpal extending into the carpometacarpal joint.

### Differential Diagnosis

▶ Bennett or Rolando fracture.

### Teaching Points

#### Etiology

▶ Both Bennett and Rolando fractures caused by axial force directed onto a partially flexed metacarpal.

#### Prognosis

▶ Bennett fractures with displacement of 1 mm or less typically associated with excellent outcomes.
▶ Rolando fracture uncommon but associated with decreased long-term grip strength and mobility. Also more difficult to treat than Bennett fracture.

### Management

#### Bennett

▶ Operative management preferred, because conservative measures associated with worse clinical outcomes. General indication for conservative management includes an articular step-off of 2 mm or less. Surgery includes open or percutaneous techniques.

#### Rolando

▶ High degree of comminution precludes operative treatment; if two large fracture fragments exist, without significant comminution, operative management is preferred.

### Further Readings

Zhang X, Shao Zhang, et al. Treatment of a Bennett fracture using tension band wiring. *J Hand Surg.* 2012;37:427–433.
Kjaer-Peterson K, Langhoff L, Anderson K. Bennett's fracture. *J Hand Surg Br.* 1990;15:58–61.
Carlsen BT, Moran SL. Thumb trauma: Bennett fractures, Rolando fractures, and ulnar collateral ligament injuries. *J Hand Surg.* 2009;34:945–952.

### History

20-year-old male status post fall from height.

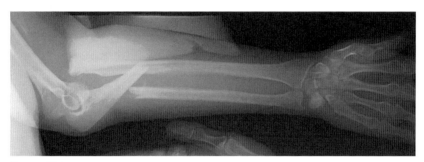

**Figure 69.1**

# Case 69  Monteggia Fracture-Dislocation

### Findings

▶ Fracture of the ulna with radial head dislocation from the capitellum
▶ Ulnar fracture usually involves the proximal one-third of the ulna
▶ Dislocation of the radial head is most frequently anterior

### Differential Diagnosis

▶ Isolated fracture of the ulna
▶ Galeazzi fracture-dislocation
▶ Anterior elbow dislocation

### Teaching Points

▶ Etiology
  ▪ Direct blow to the forearm
  ▪ Fall on an outstretched hand with forced pronation
▶ Epidemiology: Uncommon, approximately 1%–2% of all forearm fractures. Most common in adult males.
▶ Separate radiographs of the elbow and forearm are helpful in uncertain cases particularly when radial head dislocation is not obvious
▶ Bado classification based primarily on direction of radial head dislocation. Ulnar fracture angulation corresponds to direction of radial head dislocation.

### Management

▶ Usually with open reduction internal fixation

### Further Readings

Beutel BG. Monteggia fractures in pediatric and adult populations. *Orthopedics*. 2012;35(2):138–144.
Eathiraju S, Mudgal CS, Jupiter JB. Monteggia fracture-dislocations. *Hand Clin*. 2007;23(2):165–177.

# Section 6    Lower Extremity

**History**

▶ None

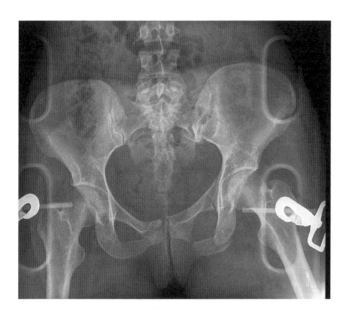

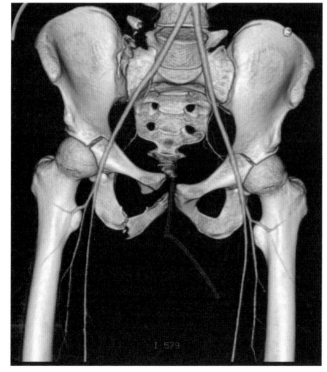

**Figures 70.1–70.2**

# Case 70 Pelvic Fracture, Anteroposterior Compression

## Findings

▶ Vertical sacral fracture with sacroiliac joint diastasis
▶ Fractures of the bilateral superior and inferior pubic rami
▶ Diastasis of the pubic symphysis
▶ Three-dimensional CT image demonstrates a similar pattern of findings, with fractures of the acetabula and transverse processes

## Teaching Points

▶ Injury occurs due to anterior or posterior forces, usually from MVA.
▶ Classified into three types
  ▪ Type I: Vertical fracture of the superior and inferior pubic rami on one or both sides, with mild widening of the pubic symphysis and/or the sacroiliac joint.
  ▪ Type II: Diastasis of the pubic symphysis and unilateral or bilateral sacroiliac joints anteriorly, with disruption of the sacrospinous, sacrotuberous, and anterior sacroiliac ligaments. Intact posterior sacroiliac ligaments. Produces an open-book type of fracture when both the iliac bones are rotated externally.
  ▪ Type III: Complete disruption of the anterior and posterior sacroiliac joints causing lateral displacement and complete separation of the iliac wing from the sacrum.
▶ Type II and III fractures are unstable. Concomitant posterior acetabular wall fracture or posterior dislocation is common, but sacral fractures are rare.
▶ Variants include bucket-handle fracture, characterized by ipsilateral fractures of the rami, with contralateral sacroiliac joint diastasis or fracture; and straddle fracture, caused by direct impact on the pubic symphysis with resultant bilateral superior and inferior pubic rami or obturator ring fractures.

## Management

▶ Treatment of associated arterial and bladder/urethral injuries.
▶ If stable, managed conservatively. Unstable fractures require pelvic stabilization and open reduction.

### Further Readings

Mirvis ES, Shanmuganathan K. *Imaging in Trauma and Critical Care.* 2nd ed. Philadelphia, Pa: Saunders, 2003.
Harris JH, Harris WH. *The Radiology of Emergency Medicine. 4th ed. Philadelphia: Lippincott, Williams & Wilkins;* 1999.
Manaster BJ, May GA, Disler DG. *Musculoskeletal imaging: the requisites,* 3rd ed. St. Louis, MO: Mosby, 2006.

## History

▸ None

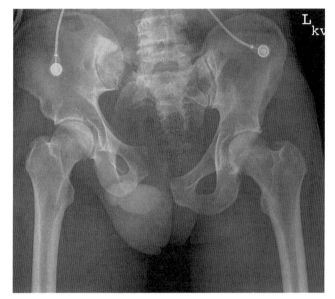

**Figure 71.1**

# Case 71  Vertical shear fracture

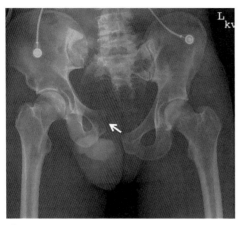 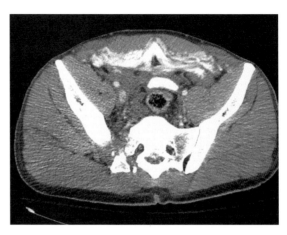

**Figures 71.2–71.3**

## Findings

▶ Superior hemipelvis displacement (right-sided on radiograph image).
▶ Sacral fractures (right-sided shown).
▶ Vertical pubic rami fractures (right-sided, arrow).
▶ Evidence of bladder and urethral injuries can be seen by contrast extravasation within the space of Retzius from extraperitoneal bladder rupture (axial CT image), with or without intraperitoneal rupture.

## Teaching Points

▶ Results from a fall from height onto the lower extremities.
▶ Superior-inferior forces cause unstable injury.
  ▪ Manifests as a vertically oriented fracture through the pubic rami and either the sacrum or sacroiliac complex. Alternatively, diastasis of the sacroiliac joint and the pubic symphysis with superior displacement of the ipsilateral hemipelvis, caused by ligamentous disruption, may be seen. Also termed a Malgaigne fracture.
  ▪ Disruption of the sacrospinous and sacrotuberous ligaments.
▶ Higher incidence of arterial injury and urethral injury in males.

## Management

▶ Control of life-threatening hemorrhage.
▶ Pelvic stabilization with external fixators followed by intraoperative fixation of the fractures.
▶ Retrograde cystogram and urethrogram to evaluate for bladder or urethral injuries.

## Further Reading

Yoon W, Kim JK, Jeong YY, et al. Pelvic arterial hemorrhage in patients with pelvic fractures: detection with contrast-enhanced CT. *RadioGraphics*. 2004;24:1591–1605.

## History

▸ None

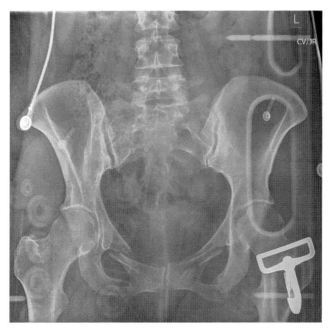

**Figure 72.1**

# Case 72  Lateral Compression Fracture

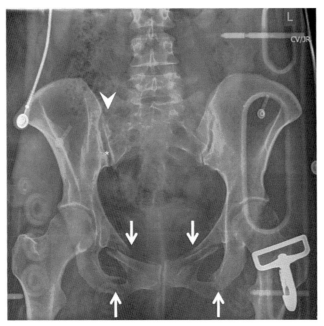

**Figure 72.2**

## Findings

▶ Horizontal pubic rami fractures (arrows).
▶ Sacral impaction fracture (arrowhead) and sacroiliac joint diastalsis (asterisk).
▶ Iliac fractures with or without rotation of hemipelvic segments (see below).

## Teaching Points

▶ Most common type of fracture from lateral impaction forces.
▶ Classified into three types.
  ▪ Type I: sacral impaction fracture at the site of the impact and horizontal fractures of unilateral or bilateral pubic rami.
  ▪ Type II: horizontal fractures of the pubic rami accompanied by either widening of the posterior sacroiliac joint and internal rotation of the anterior hemipelvic segment or fracture of the iliac wing or sacrum.
  ▪ Type III: internal rotation of the ipsilateral pelvis on the side of impact and external rotation of the contralateral hemipelvis, with disruption of the contralateral ligaments. Usually associated with ipsilateral lateral compression type I or II fracture and contralateral anteroposterior compression fracture. An unstable fracture with high risk of arterial injury.

## Management

▶ Pelvic reduction by external fixators or open reduction and internal fixation.

### Further Readings

Mirvis SE, Shanmuganathan K (eds.): *Imaging in trauma and critical care*, 2nd ed. Philadelphia, PA, W.B. Saunders, 2003.
Harris JHJ, Harris WH. *The radiology of emergency medicine*, 4th ed. Philadelphia: Lippincott Williams & Wilkins, 1999.
Manaster BJ, May DA, Disler DG. *Musculoskeletal imaging: the requisites*. 3rd ed. St Louis, Mo: Mosby, 2006.

## History

▸ None

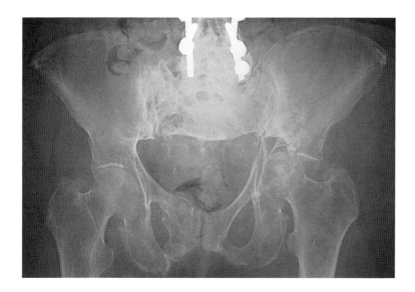

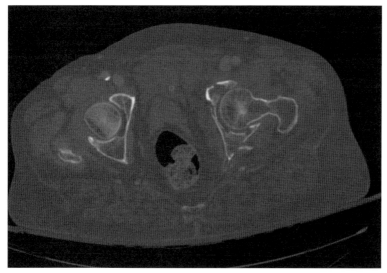

**Figures 73.1–73.2**

# Case 73  Acetabular Fracture

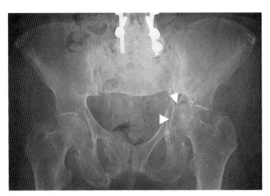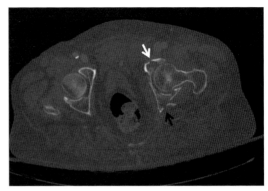

**Figures 73.3–73.4**

## Findings

▸ Radiograph and axial CT images demonstrate a complex, comminuted, both column left acetabular fracture extending into the left iliac wing (black and white arrows), and protrusion acetabula (arrow heads). Minimally displaced fractures of the left superior and inferior pubic rami and old fractures of the right superior and inferior pubic rami are also seen. The patient has undergone posterior lumbar spine fixation.

## Teaching Points

▸ Letournel's system classifies acetabular fractures into 10 major fracture patterns, of which five are simple and five are complex.
▸ Simple fracture patterns include posterior wall; posterior column (obturator ring and ilioischial line are interrupted); anterior wall; anterior column (obturator ring and iliopectineal line are interrupted with fracture of the iliac wing); and transverse acetabular fracture, which divides the acetabulum into superior and inferior halves (disrupting the ilioischial and iliopectineal lines).
▸ Complex fracture patterns include posterior column with posterior wall; transverse with posterior wall; T-type (transverse and inferior vertical fracture components); anterior column with posterior hemitransverse fracture; and both column fractures.

## Management

▸ Fractures with no or minimal displacement, or sparing of the superior acetabular dome, can be maintained conservatively with closed reduction and traction. ORIF is indicated in most displaced fractures.

Further Readings

Brandser E, Marsh JL. Acetabular fractures: easier classification with a systematic approach. *AJR Am J Roentgenol.* 1998;171:1217–1228.
Manaster BJ, May DA, Disler DG. *Musculoskeletal imaging: the requisites.* 3rd ed. St Louis, Mo: Mosby, 2006.

**History**

▶ None

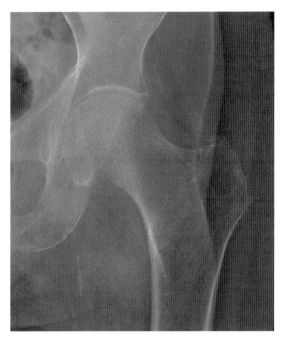

**Figure 74.1**

# Case 74   Femoral Neck Fracture

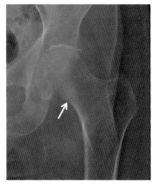 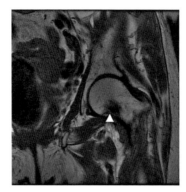 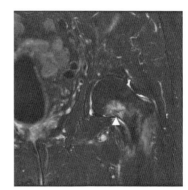

**Figures 74.2–74.4**

## Findings

▸ Subtle increased sclerosis involving the medial cortex of the left femoral neck (arrow). Corresponding coronal T1 and T2 FSE MRI images demonstrate abnormal decreased and increased signal, respectively, involving the medial cortex of the subcapital femoral neck (arrowheads).

## Differential Diagnosis

▸ Overlying marginal osteophytes could be mistaken for subcapital fracture.

## Teaching Points

▸ Two methods for classification. Divided into three types based on the site of fracture
  ▪ Subcapital: inferior to the femoral head.
  ▪ Transcervical: between the subcapital region and intertrochanteric crest.
  ▪ Basicervical: base of the femoral neck.
▸ Garden method divides the fracture into four types based on the degree of displacement
  ▪ Stage 1: incomplete fracture
  ▪ Stage 2: complete fracture without displacement
  ▪ Stage 3: complete fracture with minimal displacement
  ▪ Stage 4: complete fracture with displacement
▸ Complications, including nonunion and avascular necrosis, increase with degree of displacement.

## Management

▸ Nondisplaced fractures are treated with Knowles pin or screw fixation. Displaced fractures or patients with preexisting severe degenerative changes are treated with hip arthroplasty.

## Further Readings

Harris JHJ, Harris WH. *The radiology of emergency medicine*, 4th ed. Philadelphia: Lippincott Williams & Wilkins, 1999.
Manaster BJ, May DA, *Disler DG, Musculoskeletal imaging: the requisites*. 3rd ed. St Louis, Mo: Mosby, 2006.

# Case 75

## History

▶ None

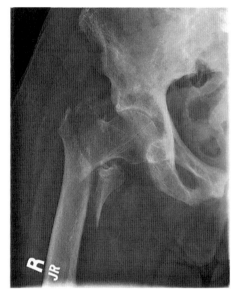
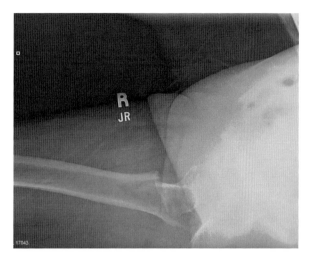

**Figures 75.1–75.2**

# Case 75  Intertrochanteric Fracture

**Findings**

▶ Intertrochanteric fracture with proximal and distal fragments and fracture of both greater and lesser trochanters.

**Teaching Points**

▶ Classified based on the number of fracture fragments as
  ▪ Two-part: Proximal and distal fragments.
  ▪ Three-part: Proximal and distal fragments and either the lesser or the greater trochanter.
  ▪ Four-part: Proximal and distal fragments, greater and lesser trochanters.
▶ Isolated greater and lesser trochanter fractures are associated with avulsion of the gluteus medius/minimus and iliopsoas muscles, respectively.

**Management**

▶ ORIF with cortical femoral plate and dynamic hip screw.

Further Readings

Harris JH, Harris WH. *The Radiology of Emergency Medicine*. 4th ed. Philadelphia: Lippincott, Williams & Wilkins; 1999.
Manaster BJ, May GA, Disler DG. *Musculoskeletal imaging: the requisites*, 3rd ed. St. Louis, MO: Mosby, 2006.

## History

▶ 55-year-old man status post motor vehicle collision with direct trauma to left knee.

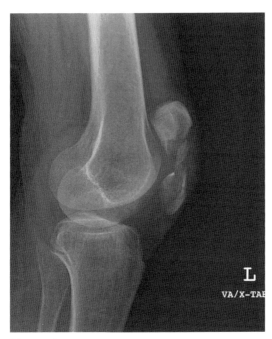

**Figure 76.1**

# Case 76  Patellar fracture

## Findings

Patellar fractures may be displaced or nondisplaced; involve the mid, lower, or upper pole; and may be comminuted, transverse, or vertical in orientation. Fractures may also be osteochondral in nature.

## Differential Diagnosis

▶ Bipartite patella
▶ Tendon rupture
▶ Patellar dislocation

## Teaching Points

▶ Mechanisms of injury include direct, indirect, and combined trauma
  ▪ Direct: Typically results from a fall or from impact against the dashboard in a motor vehicle collision. The patella is predisposed to fracture by a paucity of anterior prepatellar soft tissue and a rigid femur, posteriorly. Direct fractures are usually comminuted.
  ▪ Indirect: Occurs during jumping or unexpected rapid flexion of the knee against a fully contracted quadriceps muscle. It results from a three-point tension between the quadriceps tendon superiorly, the infrapatellar tendon inferiorly, and the femur posteriorly. Indirect fractures are usually transverse and displaced.
▶ Orientation of fracture lines includes transverse, vertical, and stellate. Vertical fracture is rare.
▶ AO Classification
  ▪ A: extra-articular—extensor mechanism avulsion
  ▪ B: partial articular—extensor mechanism intact
  ▪ C: Complete articular—disrupted extensor mechanism
▶ Patellar fracture can be mistaken with bipartite patella. However, bipartite patella is located in the upper outer quadrant, and has corticated margins.
▶ On physical examination there may be a palpable abnormality and possibly excessive extension.

## Management

Surgical intervention may be necessary.

### Further Reading

Tuong B, White J, Louis L, Cairns R, Andrews G, Forster B. Get a kick out of this: the spectrum of knee extensor mechanism injuries. *Br J Sports Med*. 2011;45:140–146.

## History

▶ None

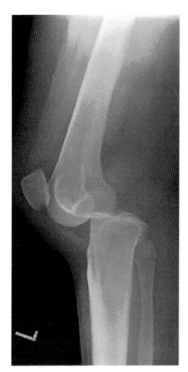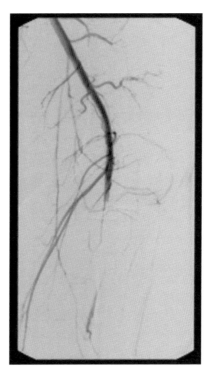

**Figures 77.1–77.2**

# Case 77  Knee Dislocation, Posterior

### Findings

▸ The tibia is posteriorly displaced relative to the distal femur (no associated fracture in this case).
▸ Direct angiography demonstrates injury to the popliteal artery with abrupt cut-off.

### Differential Diagnosis

None

### Teaching Points

▸ Occurs with high-velocity injuries, such as motor vehicle crashes, and low-velocity mechanisms, such as martial arts kicks and water skiing.
▸ Usually results in rupture of three of the four major stabilizing ligaments of the knee, although occasionally only two of the ligaments are torn.
▸ Knowledge of mechanism and physical examination findings, in addition to imaging findings, is important because dislocated knees may reduce spontaneously and may lead to missed or delayed diagnosis.
▸ CT arteriography to determine if there has been concomitant popliteal artery injury should be performed, because the incidence has been reported to be between 21% and 32% in cases of posterior knee dislocation.

### Management

▸ Most patients with multiligament knee injuries undergo surgical management; however, some patients may be best served by a nonoperative approach, with the goal of achieving good range of motion and strength and normal gait mechanics.
▸ Open vascular repair, such as direct repair with or without arteriorrhaphy, interposition replacement, and bypass graft, remains the standard of care in managing vascular injury associated with extremity trauma. Although surgical technique affects outcome, results are primarily dependent on early detection of vascular injury followed by immediate treatment.

### Further Readings

Skendzel JG, Sekiya JK, Wojtys EM. Diagnosis and management of the multiligament-injured knee. *J Orthop Sports Phys Ther*. 2012;42(3):234–42. PMID: 22383035

Halvorson JJ, Anz A, Langfitt M, et al. Vascular injury associated with extremity trauma: initial diagnosis and management. *J Am Acad Orthop Surg*. 2011;19(8):495–504. PMID: 21807917

Merritt AL, Wahl C. Initial assessment of the acute and chronic multiple-ligament injured (dislocated) knee. *Sports Med Arthrosc*. 2011;19(2):93–103. PMID: 21540706

Rajeswaran G, Williams A, Mitchell AW. Radiology and management of multiligament injuries of the knee. *Semin Musculoskelet Radiol*. 2011;15(1):42–58. PMID: 21332019

**History**

► None

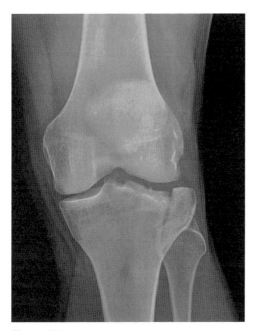

**Figure 78.1**

# Case 78   Tibial Plateau Fracture

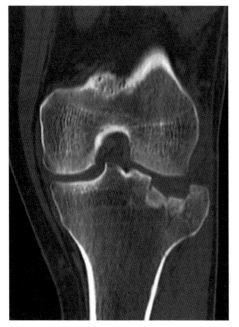 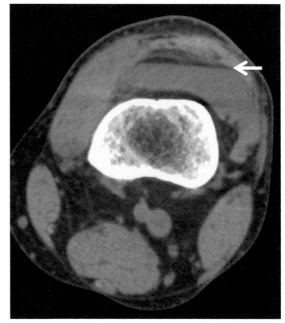

**Figures 78.2–78.3**

## Findings

▶ Fat-fluid level in the suprapatellar bursa (lipohemarthrosis) on plain radiography, best seen on cross-table lateral views.

▶ Tibial plateau fracture may be subtle on routine two-view radiography. Oblique radiography and/or CT should be considered for further evaluation in case of high suspicion.

▶ Younger patients: vertical split fracture.

▶ Older patients: depressed plateau may appear as a sclerotic line below the level of the cortex.

## Differential Diagnosis

▶ ACL tear and associated Segond fracture

▶ MCL/LCL avulsion fracture

## Teaching Points

▶ CT is better for detecting occult fractures and characterizes fracture fragments (size, depression, position, comminution), which can influence surgical management.

▶ Lateral plateau fracture more common than medial plateau.

▶ 25% are caused by motor vehicle accident; "bumper" or "fender."

▶ Schatzker and OTA/AO classification used by orthopedic surgeons to determine surgical management.

## Management

▶ Reduction and early ambulation.

▶ Immediate surgery if open fracture, neurovascular injury or compartment syndrome.

### Further Readings

Markhardt BK, Gross JM, Monu JU. Schatzker classification of tibial plateau fractures: use of CT and MR imaging improves assessment. *RadioGraphics.* 2009;29:585–597.

Computed tomography of tibial plateau fractures. *AJR Am J Roentgenol.* 1984;142(6):1181–1186.

## History

▶ None

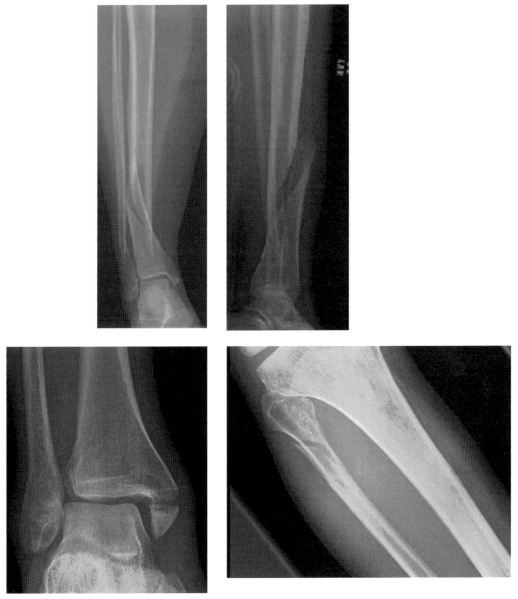

**Figures 79.1–79.4**

# Case 79  Maisonneuve Fracture

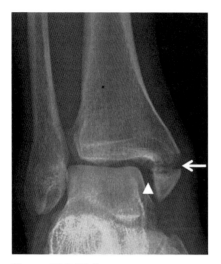 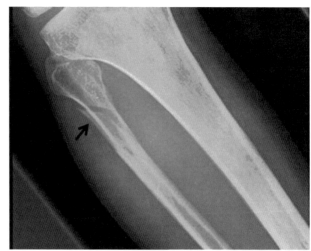

**Figures 79.5–79.6**

## Findings

### Radiography

▶ Horizontally orientated fracture through the base of the medial malleolus (white arrow)
▶ Widening of the medial clear space of the ankle mortise (arrowhead)
▶ Spiral fracture of the proximal fibula (black arrow)

## Differential Diagnosis

None

## Teaching Points

▶ Spiral fracture of the upper third of the fibula with disruption of the distal tibiofibular syndesmosis and associated injuries (e.g., fracture of the medial malleolus, fracture of the posterior malleolus, and rupture of the deltoid ligament)
▶ Fibular fracture occurs secondary to external rotation at the ankle (with the foot in either eversion or inversion)
  ▪ An eversion external rotation type of fibular fracture is associated with a nondisplaced fracture of the posterior tubercle of the tibia and always with rupture of the syndesmosis and anterior capsule of the ankle joint
▶ If an injury of the medial ankle joint is noted, namely widening of the medial clear space or an isolated medial malleolar fracture, then radiographs of the rest of the tibia and fibula are indicated

## Management

▶ Goal is to maintain a normal ankle mortise
▶ Reduction of the fibula is important, because shortening results in lateral talar displacement, which predisposes the patient to painful ankle arthrosis
▶ The tibiofibular syndesmosis is usually treated with a syndesmotic screw

## Further Readings

Hutchinson AJ, Frampton AE, Bhattacharya R. Operative fixation for complex tibial fractures. *Ann R Coll Surg Engl.* 2012;94(1):34–38. PMID: 22524923
Mashru RP, Herman MJ, Pizzutillo PD. Tibial shaft fractures in children and adolescents. *J Am Acad Orthop Surg.* 2005;13(5):345–352. PMID: 16148360

**History**

► Hindfoot trauma

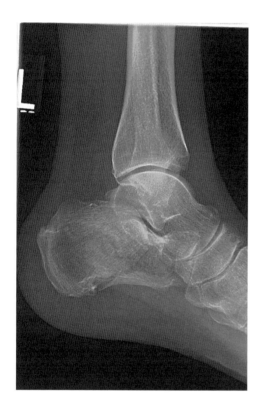
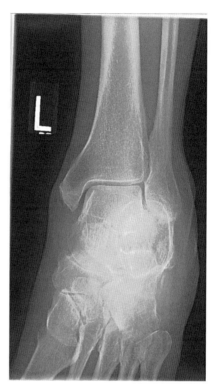
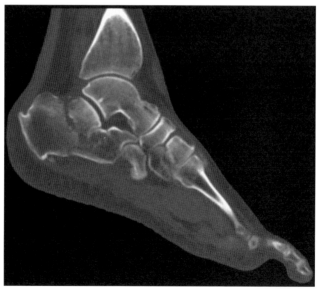

**Figures 80.1–80.3**

# Case 80  Calcaneal Fracture

### Findings

▶ Comminuted calcaneal fracture demonstrating fracture lines extending caudally and posteriorly from the angle of Gissane, and a secondary fracture line extending superiorly and posteriorly toward the superior calcaneal border

▶ Boehler angle is <20 degrees

▶ Impactions and angulation of the posterior facet is seen on CT

### Teaching Points

▶ Calcaneal fractures account for 60% of all tarsal injuries and are mostly caused by motor vehicle collisions and falls (high force compression mechanism)

▶ The angle of Boehler is an important angle obtained from a lateral radiograph
  ▪ Formed by the intersection of a line from the highest point of the posterior calcaneal tuberosity to the highest point of the posterior facet, and a second line from the latter point to the highest point of the anterior process
  ▪ An angle of Boehler less than 20 degrees indicates posterior facet collapse from an underlying calcaneal fracture

▶ Sanders system of classification is the most commonly used for intra-articular fractures (75% calcaneal fractures)
  ▪ Based on fracture lines through the posterior facet of the subtalar joint
  ▪ Type I: Nondisplaced (displacement <2 mm), regardless of number
  ▪ Type II: Single fracture line with two articular fragments
    ▪ IIA: lateral fracture line
    ▪ IIB: central fracture line
    ▪ IIC: medial fracture line
  ▪ Type III: Two fracture lines with three articular fragments
  ▪ Type IV: Comminuted (>3 fragments)

▶ Extra-articular fractures (25%) include all fractures that do not involve the posterior facet of the subtalar joint
  ▪ Type A: Anterior process of calcneus
  ▪ Type B: Body of calcaneus
  ▪ Type C: Posterior calcaneus (including posterior tuberosity and medial tubercle)

▶ Approximately 10% of affected individuals also present with compression injuries of the spine, most commonly in the thoracolumbar region between the T12 and L2 vertebrae

### Management

▶ In general, nonsurgical treatment is indicated for nondisplaced or minimally displaced closed extra-articular fractures

▶ Open reduction with internal fixation within 3 weeks after displaced intra-articular and open fractures

## History

▶ Trauma to lateral foot.

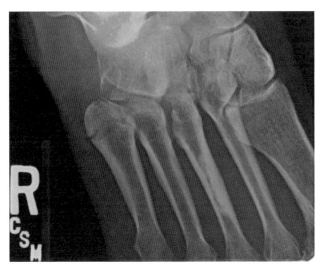 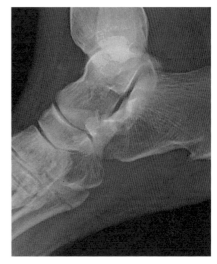

**Figures 81.1–81.2**

# Case 81  Metatarsal Fracture

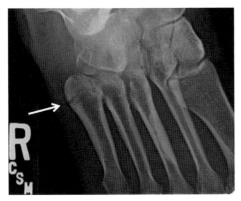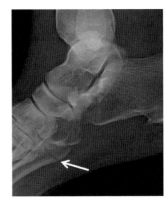

**Figures 81.3–81.4**

## Findings

▸ Transversely orientated proximal fifth metatarsal fracture extends into the cuboid-metatarsal articulation (arrows).

## Differential Diagnosis

▸ Jones fracture
▸ Stress fracture

## Teaching Points

▸ Three anatomic subgroups to proximal fifth metatarsal fractures
  ▪ Tuberosity avulsion fractures—can extend into the cuboid-metatarsal articulation)
  ▪ Fractures at the metaphyseal/diaphyseal junction, extending into but no further than the fourth/fifth intermetatarsal articulation (Jones fracture)
  ▪ Proximal diaphyseal stress fractures
▸ Avulsion fractures occur at the insertion of the peroneus brevis and lateral cord of the plantar fascia.
▸ Distinction between Jones and proximal diaphyseal fractures is often difficult but not usually necessary because the clinical outcomes are not different between the two fracture locations.
▸ Fractures of the base distal to the tuberosity can also be classified based on radiologic appearances
  ▪ Torg Type I: narrow fracture line, absent intramedullary sclerosis
  ▪ Torg type II: widening of the fracture line and evidence of intramedullary sclerosis
  ▪ Torg type III: complete obliteration of the medullary canal by sclerotic bone

## Management

▸ Nondisplaced tuberosity avulsion fractures can be treated conservatively, but surgical treatment is indicated if the fracture is displaced more than 2 mm or when there is more than 30% of the cubometatarsal joint involved.
▸ The Jones fracture is known for prolonged healing time and even nonunion.
▸ Nondisplaced or minimally displaced shaft fractures can be treated conservatively; however, screw or percutaneous K-wire fixation is indicated when the dislocation is >3–4 mm or the angulation is >10 degrees.
▸ Indication for operative treatment also depends on Torg classification
  ▪ Type I fractures are managed nonoperative
  ▪ Type II fractures can be managed nonoperative or operatively, depending on activity level
  ▪ Type III fractures have more complications and should be operated on

## Further Readings

Zwitser EW, Breederveld RS. Fractures of the fifth metatarsal: diagnosis and treatment. *Injury*. 2010;41(6):555–562. PMID: 1957053
Rammelt S, Heineck J, Zwipp H. Metatarsal fractures. *Injury*. 2004;35(suppl 2):SB77–SB86. PMID: 1531588

**History**

▸ None

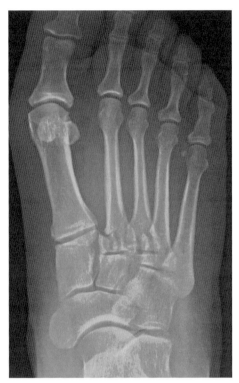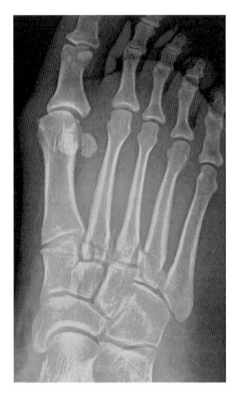

**Figures 82.1–82.2**

# Case 82  Lisfranc Injury

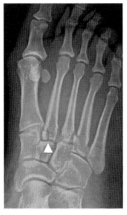 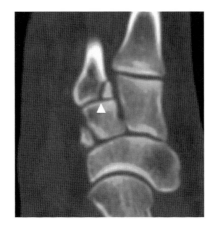 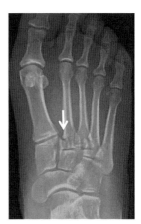

**Figures 82.3–82.5**

## Findings

▶ Malalignment of the medial border of the second metatarsal with the medial border of the middle cuneiform (arrow).

▶ Mildly displaced intra-articular fracture of the medial base of the second metatarsal (arrowheads) occurs at the insertion of the Lisfranc ligament.

## Differential Diagnosis

None

## Teaching Points

▶ Fracture dislocation of the tarsometatarsal (Lisfranc) joint is an uncommon foot injury, and up to one-third is missed on initial presentation.

▶ Three types of injury
- Type A: Total incongruity of the tarsometatarsal joint. Displacement is in one plane, which can be sagittal, coronal, or combined.
- Type B: Partial incongruity of the joint, which may be medial or lateral.
  - Medial displacement affects the first metatarsal, either isolated or combined with the second, third, or fourth metatarsal
  - With lateral displacement the first metatarsal is unaffected.
- Type C (divergent-type): Partial or total incongruity may be present. The first metatarsal is displaced medially and any of the other metatarsals could be displaced laterally.

▶ On AP view, diastasis of >2 mm between the base of the first and second metatarsal suggests a Lisfranc injury.

▶ On lateral view, the superior border of the base of the first metatarsal should align with the superior border of the medial cuneiform.

▶ On oblique view, the medial border of the fourth metatarsal should align with the medial border of the cuboid.

▶ The "fleck" sign on AP view is pathognomonic for a Lisfranc injury and represents an avulsion fracture of the base of the second metatarsal or medial cuneiform resulting from traction of the Lisfranc ligament. It is radiologically evident in 90% of the patients with a Lisfranc fracture.

## Management

▶ Mild sprains to the Lisfranc joint that are anatomically stable and nondisplaced are treated with immobilization.

▶ Displaced or unstable Lisfranc injuries usually undergo reduction (closed or open) and operative fixation.

Further Reading

Kalia V, Fishman EK, Carrino JA, Fayad LM. Epidemiology, imaging, and treatment of Lisfranc fracture-dislocations revisited. *Skeletal Radiol.* 2012;41(2):129–136. PMID: 21431438

## History

▶ 14-year-old boy developed right knee pain while playing basketball.

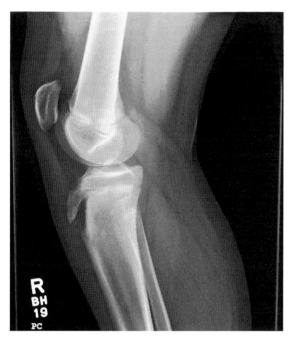

**Figure 83.1**

# Case 83  Tibial Tubercle Avulsion Fracture

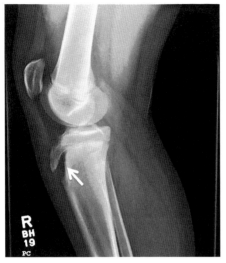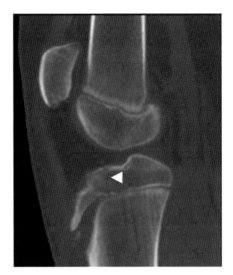

**Figures 83.2–83.3**

## Findings

Avulsion fracture of the tibial tubercle (arrow) is seen with patella alta and intra-articular extent through the epiphysis (arrowhead).

## Differential Diagnosis

▶ Osgood-Schlatter disease (chronic, irregular ossification of the tibial tubercle).
▶ Anatomic variant of the tibial tubercle.

## Teaching Points

▶ Uncommon fracture, teenage males more than females.
▶ Secondary to quadricpes contraction against a fixed lower leg or anterior blow to lower leg during quadriceps contraction.
▶ Three types
  ▪ Type I (most common)
    ▪ IA: Incomplete separation of fragment from metaphysis
    ▪ IB: Complete separation
  ▪ Type II: Tubercle epiphysis lifted anteriorly and proximally
    ▪ IIA: Single fracture
    ▪ IIB: Comminuted
  ▪ Type III: Fracture extends through the epiphysis into the joint space
    ▪ IIIA: Single fracture
    ▪ IIIB: Comminuted, displaced fragments

## Management

▶ Type I: Typically ORIF if >5 mm of asymmetric displacement of patella compared with unaffected limb on extension lateral radiograph
▶ Type II and III: Usually requires ORIF
▶ Type III: High incidence of compartment syndrome; consider prophylactic fasciotomy

## Further Readings

Dupuis CS, et al. Injuries and conditions of the extensor mechanism of the pediatric knee. *RadioGraphics*. 2009;29:877–886.
Chow SP, Lam JJ, Leong JCY. Fracture of the tibial tubercle in the adolescent. *J Bone Joint Surg*. 1990;72(2):231–234.
Ogden JA, Tross RB, Murphy MJ. Fractures of the tibial tuberosity in adolescents. *J Bone Joint Surg*. 1980;62(2):205–215.

## History

► None

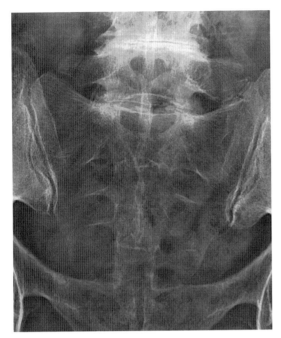

**Figure 84.1**

# Case 84  Sacral Fracture

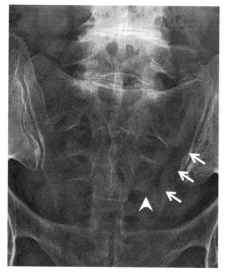
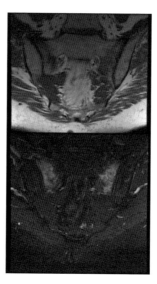

**Figures 84.2–84.3**

## Findings

▶ Fracture lucency (arrows) and disruption of the sacral arcuate lines (arrowhead) indicate the presence of fracture.

▶ Hypointense T1 and hyperintense T2 linear abnormalities are MRI findings consistent with insufficiency fractures.

## Diagnosis

Sacral fracture

## Differential Diagnosis

Pelvic fractures.

## Teaching Points

▶ Denis classification of sacral fractures
 ▪ Zone 1: Fracture occurs lateral to the sacral foramina and may cause injury to the L5 nerve root in 6% of cases.
 ▪ Zone 2: Fracture involves one or more of the sacral foramina and may lead to unilateral lumbar or sacral neuropathies. The fracture may extend to Zone 1.
 ▪ Zone 3: Fracture involves the central sacral canal and may extend to involve the other two zones. Bilateral neurologic deficits can occur, as well as bowel and bladder incontinence.
▶ Sacral insufficiency fracture
 ▪ Seen with osteoporosis or after radiation therapy. These fractures are often radiographically occult.
 ▪ Vertical, mixed sclerotic, and lucent lines along the sacral wings if the fracture is unilateral. If bilateral, a horizontal line at the level of the S2 or S3 sacral foramina produces the classic Honda sign.
 ▪ Best diagnosed on CT, MRI, or radionuclide bone scans.

## Management

▶ Usually conservative. ORIF is reserved for sacral fractures with pelvic instability and neurological deficits.

## Further Readings

Diel J, Ortiz O, Losada RA. The sacrum: pathologic spectrum, multimodality imaging, and subspecialty approach. *RadioGraphics*. 2001;21:83–104.
Manaster BJ, May DA, Disler DG. *Musculoskeletal imaging: the requisites.* 3rd ed. St Louis, Mo: Mosby, 2006.

## History

▶ None

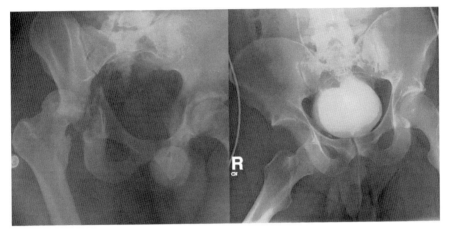

**Figure 85.1**

# Case 85   Hip Dislocation

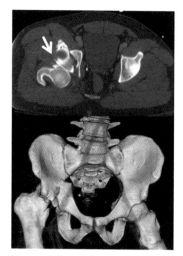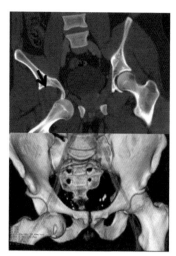

**Figures 85.2–85.3**

## Findings

▶ Posterior hip dislocation (white arrow) with associated acetabular fracture.

▶ Inferior (obturator) type anterior hip dislocation (black arrow).

## Diagnosis

Hip dislocation

## Teaching Points

▶ Posterior hip dislocation is more common than anterior dislocation.
- Clinically, the limb is shortened, adducted, extended, and internally rotated
- Femoral head is posteriorly and superiorly positioned with respect to the acetabulum, and the femur is internally rotated with greater trochanter in profile and lesser trochanter being obscured
- Associated with fracture of the posterior acetabular wall

▶ Anterior dislocation is uncommon and occurs with forced abduction and external rotation. Divided in to two types.
- Inferior (obturator) dislocation occurs with hip flexion, with the femoral head positioned anteriorly and medially over the obturator foramen
- Superior dislocation occurs with extension of the femur with the femoral head positioned superiorly and either medial or lateral to the acetabulum
- Can be confused with posterior dislocation; differentiate by external rotation (lesser trochanter in profile) with anterior dislocation and internal rotation (lesser trochanter obscured) with posterior dislocation
- Important to distinguish anterior from posterior dislocation because failure of reduction may result if misdiagnosed
- Associated with fractures of the acetabulum, femoral head, anterior superior iliac spine, and greater trochanter

▶ Complications of hip dislocation include avascular necrosis, if not reduced in a timely manner, and osteoarthritis.

## Management

▶ Closed reduction. Open reduction should be performed if closed reduction is unsuccessful, if there are associated complex fractures, if bony fragments remain in the joint space, or the joint remains unstable.

### Further Readings

Erb RE, Steele JR, Nance EP Jr, et al. Traumatic anterior dislocation of the hip: spectrum of plain film and CT findings. *AJR Am J Roentgenol.* 1995;65(5):1215–1219.

Manaster BJ, May DA, Disler DG. *Musculoskeletal imaging: the requisites.* 3rd ed. St Louis, Mo: Mosby, 2006.

**History**

▸ None

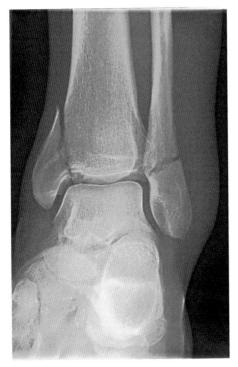

**Figure 86.1**

# Case 86  Ankle fracture

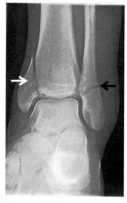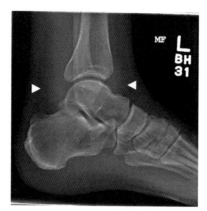

**Figures 86.2–86.3**

## Findings

▶ Oblique, vertically oriented medial malleolus fracture (white arrow).
▶ Horizontal lateral malleolus fracture (black arrow) at the level of the tibial plafond.
▶ Soft tissue swelling with tibiotalar joint effusion (arrowheads).
▶ Mortise symmetry preserved.

## Diagnosis

Bimalleolar ankle fracture. Likely inversion-type caused by fracture morphology.

## Differential diagnosis

None

## Teaching Points

▶ Two common classification schemes
  ▪ Danis-Weber classification: type A, fibular fracture below the syndesmosis; type B, fibular fracture at the level of the syndesmosis; type C, fibular fracture above the syndesmosis.
  ▪ Lauge-Hansen classification: 1. Supination-external rotation (SE) caused by external rotation of an inverted foot; 2. Pronation-external rotation caused by external rotation of an everted foot; 3. Supination-adduction (pure inversion); 4. Pronation-abduction (pure eversion).
▶ Lauge-Hansen SE injuries account for nearly two-thirds of all ankle fractures, and are disproportionately associated with low-energy trauma, older individuals, and females.
▶ SE injury has four stages
  ▪ First: Anterior tibiofibular ligament rupture
  ▪ Second: Spiral or oblique lateral malleolus fracture
  ▪ Third: Posterior tibiofibular ligament rupture or avulsion (posterior malleolar fragment)
  ▪ Fourth: Deltoid ligament rupture or avulsion (medial malleolar fragment)

## Management

▶ Indications for operative treatment: Unstable Weber B fracture; >5 mm of medial clear space on static or stress radiograph.
▶ Usually open reduction and internal fixation with plate and screw constructs along the distal fibula, and syndesmotic screws.

### Further Readings

Okanobo H, Khurana B, Sheehan S, Duran-Mendicuti A, Arianjam A, Ledbetter S. Simplified diagnostic algorithm for Lauge-Hansen classification of ankle injuries. *RadioGraphics*. 2012;32(2):E71–E84. PMID: 22411951
Mandi DM. Ankle fractures. *Clin Podiatr Med Surg*. 2012;29(2):155–186, vii. PMID: 22424483

# Part II    Nontrauma

# Section 1    Brain

## History

▶ 44-year-old male who had an upper respiratory tract infection for weeks before developing a headache and fever to 104.8 °F.

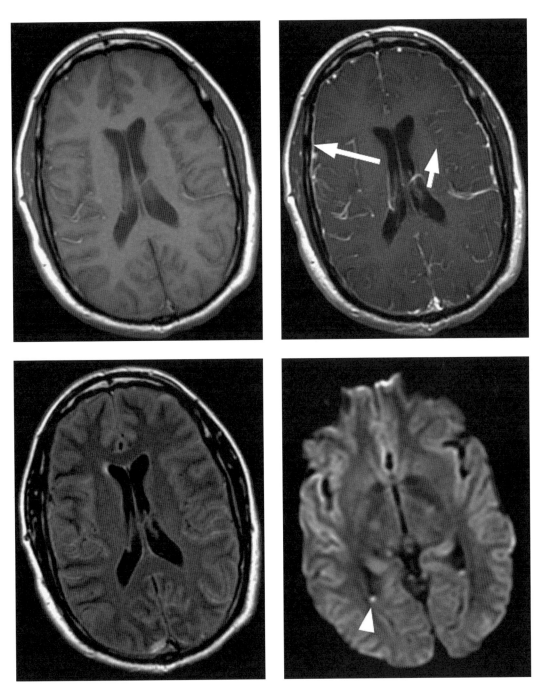

**Figures 87.1–87.4**

# Case 87  Meningitis

## Findings

▶ Diffuse pachymeningeal enhancement (long arrow) and scattered leptomeningeal enhancement (short arrow)
▶ Diffuse sulcal hyperintensity on FLAIR images
▶ Diffuse cerebral cortical T2 hyperintensity (FLAIR and DWI images)
▶ Mild disproportionate prominence of the ventricles relative to the sulci concerning for early hydrocephalus
▶ Layering DWI-hyperintensity, representing pus, in the lateral ventricles (arrowhead)

## Differential Diagnosis

▶ Bacterial infection: *Streptococcus, Escherichia coli, Neisseria, Mycobacterium tuberculosis, Borrelia, Haemophilus*
▶ Viral infection: Herpes simplex virus, varicella zoster virus, West Nile virus, enterovirus
▶ Neoplastic meningitis: Breast cancer, lung cancer, melanoma
▶ Inflammatory: Idiopathic hypertrophic cranial pachymeningitis, rheumatoid, sarcoid
▶ Toxic: NSAIDs, antibiotics

## Pathophysiology

▶ Meningitis results from irritation of the pachymeninges and/or the leptomeninges
▶ The spectrum of infection differs markedly between children and adults
▶ Widespread use of vaccines against *Haemophilus, Streptococcus*, and *Neisseria* has altered the epidemiology of meningitis
▶ Infection may spread from an adjacent space, such as sinuses, or be introduced with penetrating trauma, including surgery
▶ Chronic sequelae of meningitis may include cognitive deficits, epilepsy, and cranial nerve injury

## Clinical Presentation

▶ Can vary widely, even with a specific pathogen
▶ Headache, neck stiffness, and fever may be early symptoms of bacterial meningitis, followed by photophobia, confusion, and decreased consciousness
▶ Kernig and Brudzinski signs may be variably present in bacterial meningitis, and are not highly sensitive

## Teaching Points

▶ Imaging findings of meningitis are nonspecific, and may evoke a broad differential
▶ The differential may be substantially narrowed by consideration of the clinical presentation (e.g., signs of infection and meningismus) and patient demographics (e.g., age and risk factors, such as known infections, exposures, or malignancies)

## Management

▶ Lumbar puncture for CSF analysis can provide evidence of bacterial meningitis (elevated protein, decreased glucose, leukocytosis) and provide a culture specimen to identify the specific pathogen
▶ Head imaging to evaluate for elevated intracranial pressure or cerebellar tonsillar herniation is not typically warranted before lumbar puncture in the absence of clinical signs concerning for elevated intracranial pressure, such as decreased consciousness; pupil, gaze, or respiratory abnormalities; seizure; or papilledema

## History

► 55-year-old woman with fever, headache, and irritability.

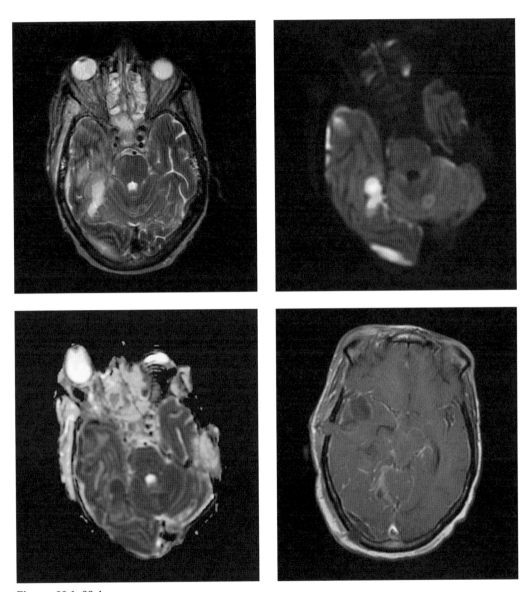

**Figures 88.1–88.4**

# Case 88  Subdural Empyema

## Findings

▸ Typically a peripherally enhancing extra-axial fluid collection, demonstrating T1 dark signal, T2/FLAIR bright signal, and restricted diffusion
▸ Similar to any subdural collections, subdural empyemas does not cross midline and is crescentic in shape

## Differential Diagnosis

▸ Sterile subdural collection (effusion), chronic subdural hematoma

## Teaching Points

▸ Etiology: Meningitis, hematogenous spread, direct extension from brain or extracranial source (such as from paranasal sinuses or mastoiditis), and complications after surgery
▸ Presentation: Fever, headache, irritability, vomiting, seizures, altered mental status, photophobia
▸ Complications: Cerebritis, cerebral abscess, and venous or arterial infarction
▸ Other pearls
  ▪ In postoperative patients, DWI does not demonstrate restricted diffusion in approximately 30% of patients (high false-negative rate); therefore, must have high clinical suspicion for subdural infection in postoperative setting even if DWI is negative
  ▪ Peripheral enhancement usually more marked in empyemas than in chronic subdural hematomas
  ▪ Blood degradation products may demonstrate restricted diffusion in postoperative patients, confounding the picture

## Management

▸ Surgical drainage and antibiotics

## Further Readings

Farrell CJ, Hoh BL, Pisculli ML, et al. Limitations of diffusion-weighted imaging in the diagnosis of postoperative infections. *Neurosurgery.* 2008;62:577–583.

Grossman RI, Yousem DM. *The Requisites: Neuroradiology.* Philadelphia: Elsevier; 2003.

Sinclair AG, Scoffings DJ. Imaging the post-operative cranium. *RadioGraphics.* 2010;30:461–482.

Wong AM, Zimmerman RA, Simon EM, et al. Diffusion-weighted MR imaging of subdural empyemas in children. *Am J Neuroradiol.* 2004;25:1016–1021.

## History

▶ 60-year-old male patient with fever and altered mental status.

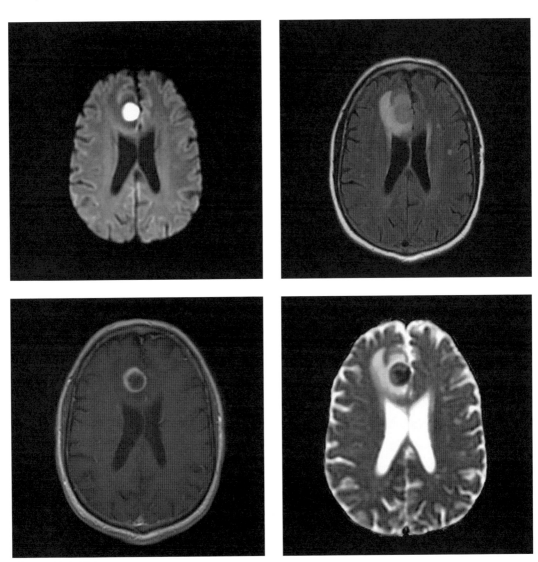

**Figures 89.1–89.4**

# Case 89   Cerebral Abscess

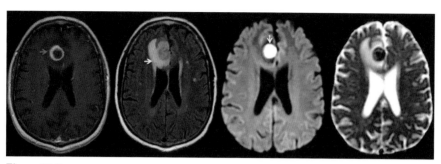

**Figure 89.5**

## Findings

### CT

▸ Complete ring enhancing lesion with surrounding areas of low attenuation (representing vasogenic edema).

### MRI

▸ Brain abscesses typically present as complete ring enhancing lesions (blue arrow) with surrounding T2 hyperintense areas of edema (light green arrow). The ring enhancing lesion has a smooth wall that is often thinner along its medial margin and it may have smaller "satellite" lesions.

▸ Diffusion weighted images demonstrate central restricted diffusion secondary to purulent material (yellow arrow). Lack of restricted diffusion is unusual for a pyogenic abscess but can be seen, particularly after partial treatment with antibiotics. Fungal and tuberculous abscesses may also lack internal restricted diffusion.

## Differential Diagnosis

▸ Primary or secondary cerebral neoplasm with central necrosis
▸ Cystic parasitic diseases
▸ Resolving hematoma

## Teaching Points

▸ A cerebral abscess is a focal infection of the brain parenchyma produced by bacteria, fungi, or mycobacteria, resulting in the development of a collection of purulent material surrounded by a discrete capsule. A focal region of cerebritis often precedes formation of a brain abscess.

▸ Cerebral abscesses typically present as intracerebral complete ring enhancing lesions with central restricted diffusion. Lack of internal restricted diffusion does not exclude a cerebral abscess.

## Management

▸ Antimicrobial and medical treatment for small abscesses. Larger abscesses, particularly with local mass effect, usually require surgical evacuation.

### Further Readings

Hughes DC, Raghavan A, Mordekar SR, Griffiths PD, Connolly DJA. Role of imaging in the diagnosis of acute bacterial meningitis and its complications. *Postgrad Med J.* 2010;86(1018):478–485.

Kastrup O, Wanke I, Maschke M. Neuroimaging of infections of the central nervous system. *Semin Neurol.* 2008;28(4):511–522.

## History

▸ 48-year-old male with HIV (viral load of 900,000 copies/ml) presents with confusion, aphasia, and right-sided weakness.

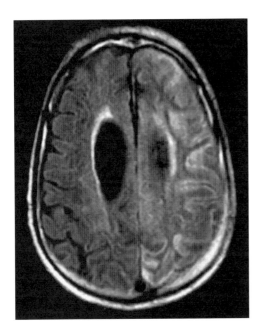
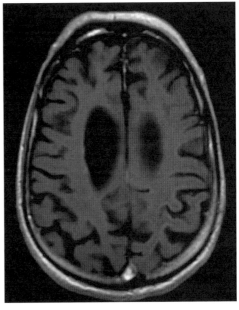
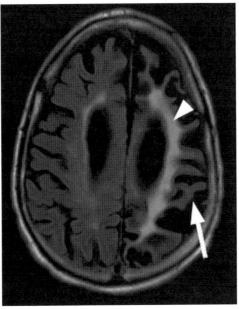

**Figures 90.1–90.3**

# Case 90   Encephalitis

## Findings

- Findings of HIV encephalitis
- Abnormal T2 hyperintensity in the cerebral hemispheres, more pronounced within the cortex and asymmetrically much greater in the left cerebral hemisphere than the right
- No significant enhancement on postcontrast images
- Patchy restricted diffusion in the right cerebral hemisphere, including involvement of the left perirolandic cortex
- T1 and T2 hyperintense subdural collections overlying the cerebral hemispheres, also more pronounced on the left than the right
- Follow-up head MRI 2.5 years later demonstrates severe atrophy (arrow) and confluent leukoencephalopathy (arrowhead) asymmetrically involving the left cerebral hemisphere

## Clinical Presentation

- Focal neurologic deficits may be present corresponding to regions of greatest brain parenchymal abnormality (e.g., right-sided weakness related to involvement of the left perirolandic region in this patient)
- Global neurologic deficits may be present, such as decreased consciousness, coma, and seizure
- Signs and symptoms of infection, such as fever, nausea, and malaise, are common
- Onset may be insidious or acute

## Pathophysiology

- Inflammatory process in the brain parenchyma that may be caused by viral, bacterial, autoimmune, or other inflammatory etiologies
- Viral: Herpes simplex virus, HIV, West Nile virus, VZV, CMV, measles, and others
- Bacterial and fungal (rare): Mycoplasma streptococcus; cryptococcus
- Autoantibody: Anti-NMDA, Hashimoto encephalitis, paraneoplastic syndromes
- Inflammatory: Acute disseminated encephalomyelitis, progressive multifocal leukoencephalopathy

## Teaching Points

- Clinical presentations of encephalitis frequently include idiosyncratic neurologic symptoms that often defy simple syndromic classification
- Imaging findings may be nonspecific and atypical
- Correlation with patient demographic data and known risk factors may be helpful to produce a focused differential
- Electroencephalography abnormalities may correlate with areas of encephalitis-affected brain tissue

## Management

- Supportive care: Directed toward maintenance of physiologic integrity in the brain. Therapies may include antiseizure medications; sedatives, including barbiturates, to prevent excitotoxic neuronal injury; and nonsteroidal anti-inflammatory drugs
- Directed therapy targeted to a demonstrated etiology, such as antiviral and other antibiotic therapies; intravenous immunoglobulin; plasmapheresis; and glucocorticoids

## History

▶ 8-year-old male patient with cough, fever, and weakness.

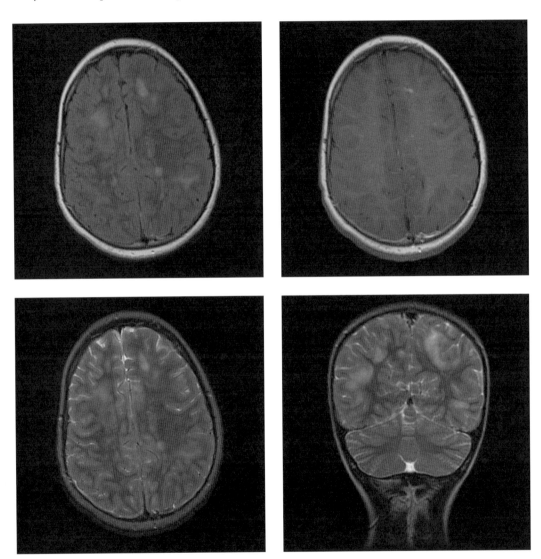

**Figures 91.1–91.4**

# Case 91  Acute Disseminated Encephalomyelitis

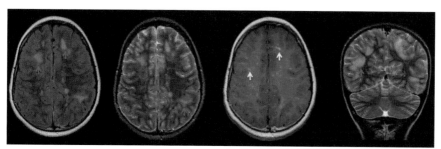

**Figure 91.5**

## Findings

### MRI

▶ Large asymmetrical white matter lesions (blue arrows) with variable enhancement (yellow arrows) and local mass effect, often involving gray matter structures, brainstem, and optic nerves.

▶ Abnormal T2 hyperintense signal and enhancement in the spinal cord.

## Differential Diagnosis

▶ Multiple sclerosis

▶ Infectious encephalomyelitis

▶ Mitochondrial disorders

▶ Neoplastic disorders, including lymphoma/leukemia and gliomas

## Teaching Points

▶ Clinical presentation: Acute disseminated encephalomyelitis is typically described as a monophasic demyelinating disorder affecting the brain and spinal cord often preceded by a viral infection or vaccination. Clinically, there is often evidence of CSF pleocytosis and encephalopathy.

▶ Clinical evolution: Follow-up imaging demonstrates marked or complete resolution of the lesions. Cases of multiphasic or recurrent acute disseminated encephalomyelitis have also been described but are considered unusual.

## Management

▶ Treatment typically consists of IV and/or oral steroids. Steroid-resistant cases are often treated with IVIg or plasmapheresis.

## Further Readings

Lim T. Neuroimaging in postinfectious demyelination and nutritional disorders of the central nervous system. *Neuroimaging Clinics N Am.* 21(4):843–858.

Parrish JB, Yeh AEA. Acuted disseminated encephalomyelitis. *Adv Exp Med Biol.* 724:1–14.

Wender M. Acute disseminated encephalomyelitis (ADEM). *J Neuroimmunol.* 231(1):92–99.

Zettl UK, Stüve O, Patejdl R. Immune-mediated CNS diseases: a review on nosological classification and clinical features. *Autoimmun Rev.* 11(3):167–173.

## History

▶ A 51-year-old woman with acute onset of severe headache.

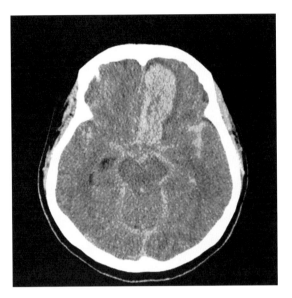 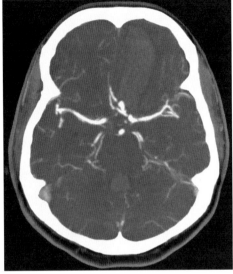

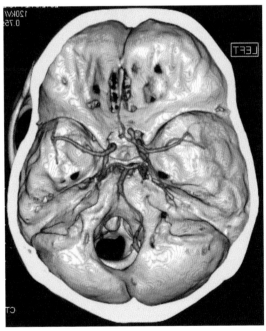

**Figures 92.1–92.3**

# Case 92   Aneurysm hemorrhage

## Findings

### CT/CTA

▷ Hyperattenuation, consistent with hemorrhage, in the basal subarachnoid spaces not limited to the perimesencephalic cisterns. Aneurysms can also bleed into the brain parenchyma, subdural space, and ventricles.

▷ An aneurysm can be seen on an unenhanced CT scan as a round or oval hyperattenuating lesion arising from a vessel.

▷ Avid enhancement of the aneurysm in the arterial phase after contrast administration.

### MR/MRA

▷ Acute subarachnoid hemorrhage: isointense signal on T1WI, and high signal intensity on T2WI and FLAIR weighted images; there may be little to no susceptibility on T2* images.

▷ Flow void of aneurysm contiguous with the parent vessel most apparent on T2WI and proton density-weighted images.

▷ Partially thrombosed aneurysms have a lamellated appearance on T2WI.

▷ Flow-related enhancement in aneurysm on MRA.

▷ Aneurysm wall well appreciated on this technique.

### Catheter Angiography

▷ Focal, saccular, dilatation of the artery with opacification on the arterial phase.

▷ Morphology of aneurysm, relation of aneurysm neck to sac, and arterial origin equally appreciated on CTA and DSA.

## Differential Diagnosis

▷ Subarachnoid hemorrhage
  ▪ Trauma
  ▪ Perimesencephalic venous hemorrhage (nonaneurysmal subarachnoid hemorrhage)
  ▪ Parenchymal hematoma that dissects into subarachnoid space
  ▪ AVM or AVF
  ▪ Bleeding tumor
  ▪ Coagulopathy
  ▪ Vasculitis
  ▪ Amyloid angiopathy
▷ Intracranial aneurysm
  ▪ Saccular aneurysms
  ▪ Fusiform aneurysms
  ▪ Mycotic aneurysms
  ▪ Oncotic aneurysms
  ▪ Aneurysms associated with AVM

## Teaching Points

▷ Quantity and pattern of blood clot on noncontrast CT may be helpful for locating a ruptured aneurysm.

▷ Aneurysms that rupture most commonly are anterior communicating, posterior communicating, middle cerebral artery bifurcation, and basilar tip aneurysms.

▷ Annual risk of rupture of aneurysms <10 mm and >10 mm is 0.7% and 4%, respectively. The risk is also higher among women, symptomatic aneurysms, aneurysms in the posterior circulation, aneurysms with a height to neck ratio of >1.6, and aneurysms that are lobulated.

## Management

▷ Endovascular coiling
▷ Surgical clipping

**History**

▸ None

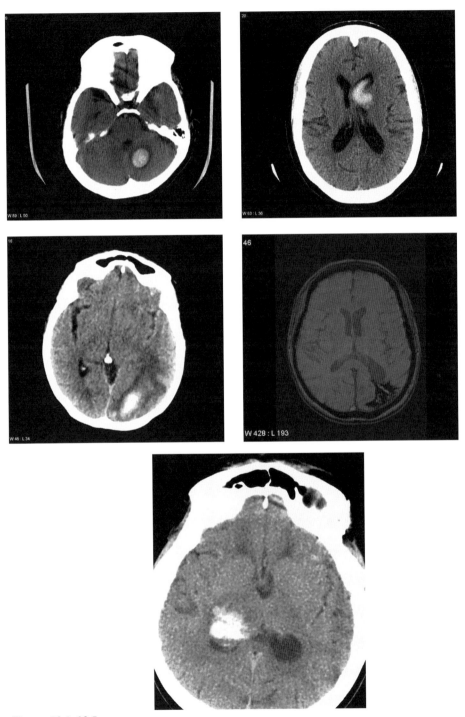

**Figures 93.1–93.5**

# Case 93  Hypertensive Intracerebral Hemorrhage

## Findings

### MRI

▶ Depending on the acuteness of the hemorrhage, the signal on T1WI and T2WI differs.

▶ Hyperacute lesions show low signal on T1 and high signal on T2.

▶ Subacute lesions show high signal on T1 and low signal on T2.

▶ Chronic lesions show low signal on T1WI and T2WI.

### NCCT

▶ Morphology
  ▪ Parenchymal hyperdense lesion, with HU between 40 and 90. These lesions commonly produce mass affect and peripheral hypoattenuation representing vasogenic edema.

▶ Common locations
  ▪ Putamen
  ▪ Thalamus
  ▪ Cerebellar and brainstem
  ▪ Lobar

## Teaching Points

▶ Thalamic hemorrhages usually drain into the ventricles.

▶ Ventricular hemorrhage is associated with poor prognosis.

▶ Mortality increases proportionally to the size of the hemorrhage.

▶ "Spot sign" predicts hematoma expansion and mortality.

## Management

▶ Intensive care has increased survival of patients with ICH.

▶ Blood pressure control.

▶ Correction of procoagulant factors.

▶ Surgical evacuation in small and superficial hemorrhage has demonstrated improved clinical outcome.

## Further Readings

Qureshi AI, Mendelow AD, Hanley DF. Intracerebral haemorrhage. *Lancet*. 20099;373(9675):1632–1644.

Chen ST, Chen SD, Hsu CY, Hogan EL. Progression of hypertensive intracerebral hemorrhage. *Neurology*. 1989;39(11):1509–1514.

Broderick JP, Brott TG, Duldner JE, Tomsick T, Huster G. Volume of intracerebral hemorrhage. A powerful and easy-to-use predictor of 30-day mortality. *Stroke*. 1993;24(7):987–993.

Delgado Almandoz JE, Yoo AJ, Stone MJ, et al. The spot sign score in primary intracerebral hemorrhage identifies patients at highest risk of in-hospital mortality and poor outcome among survivors. *Stroke*. 2010 Jan;41(1):54–60.

Goldstein JN, Fazen LE, Snider R, et al. Contrast extravasation on CT angiography predicts hematoma expansion in intracerebral hemorrhage. *Neurology*. 2007;68(12):889–894.

## History

▸ 31-year-old woman with acute right-sided weakness.

▸ Angiographic image courtesy of Drs. Chai Kobkitsuksakul and Pakorn Jiarakongmun

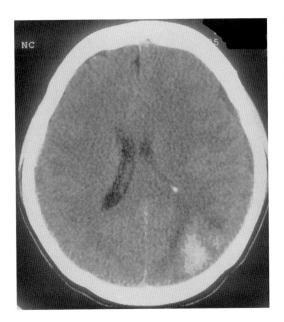
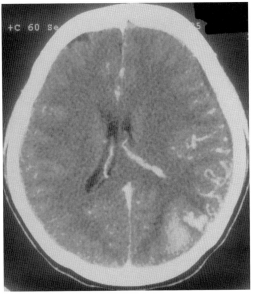
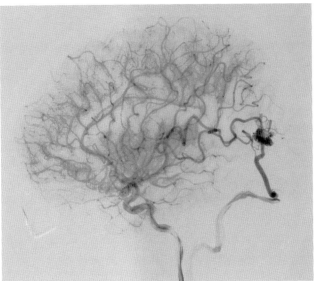

**Figures 94.1–94.3**

# Case 94 Bleeding Brain Arteriovenous Malformation

## Findings

### CT/CTA

- Hyperdense tangle of vessels ("nidus") with/without calcification
- Enlarged feeding arteries and draining cerebral veins
- Lack of mass effect unless secondary to hemorrhage
- Bleeding may occur in the brain parenchyma, subarachnoid space, or ventricles
- Localized brain atrophy

### MR/MRA

- Nidus of flow voids best appreciated on T2W and proton density-weighted images
- T2 hyperintense adjacent brain tissue caused by chronic ischemia and gliosis (steal phenomenon)
- Flow-related enhancement in feeding arteries, nidus, and draining veins

### Catheter Angiography

- Tangle of vessels between enlarged arterial feeders and draining veins
- Aneurysms of the arterial feeders, within the nidus and anywhere in the circle of Willis
- Venous stenoses in the draining veins
- An acute hematoma can obscure an AVM

## Differential Diagnosis for Hemorrhage with Abnormal Vessels

- Hemorrhagic tumor
- Dural arteriovenous fistula
- Aneurysm with parenchymal hemorrhage

## Teaching Points

- Brain AVM typically comes to attention in young adults before the age of 40 with slight male predominance.
- Most frequent clinical presentation is intracranial hemorrhage (50% of cases). AVM may bleed into brain parenchyma, subarachnoid space, or ventricles.
- Spetzler-Martin grading system categorizes AVM on the basis of
  - Size
    - 1: small, maximum diameter <3 cm
    - 2: medium, diameter 3–6 cm
    - 3: large, diameter >6 cm
  - Pattern of venous drainage
    - 0: superficial only
    - 1: any component of deep venous drainage
  - Neurologic eloquence of adjacent brain
    - 0: noneloquent areas
    - 1: eloquent areas—sensorimotor, language, and visual cortex; hypothalamus and thalamus; internal capsule; brainstem; cerebellar peduncles; and deep cerebellar nuclei
    - Patients are subjected to lifelong risk of repeated hemorrhages.
    - Multiple AVMs occur in hereditary hemorrhagic telangiectasia and Wyburn-Mason syndromes

## Management

- Surgery for AVM removal
- Radiation therapy
- Partial endovascular occlusion followed by surgery or radiation therapy

## History

▸ 66-year-old female presents with acute onset of global aphasia and right hemiparesis.

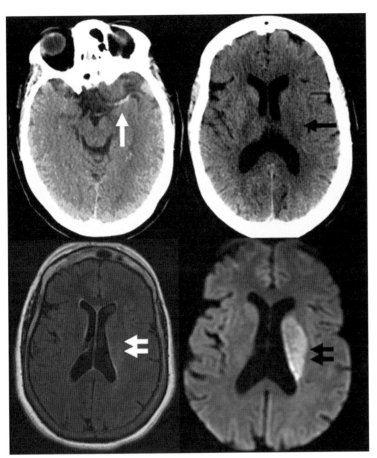

**Figure 95.1**

# Case 95  Acute Stroke

### Findings

- ▶ Noncontrast head CT in brain windows demonstrates a hyperdense left middle cerebral artery (white arrow), indicative of acute thrombus within the vessel.
- ▶ Noncontrast head CT in narrower windows demonstrates subtle hypodensity and loss of the gray-white matter differentiation in the left lentiform nucleus, caudate nucleus, and upper internal capsule (black arrow).
- ▶ CTA MIP demonstrates a left M1 occlusion.
- ▶ Axial FLAIR image demonstrates slightly increased signal within the same region (double white arrows).
- ▶ DWI image demonstrates restricted diffusion within the same region (double black arrows).
- ▶ Mean transit time map identifies prolonged transit time in a region much larger than that identified by restricted diffusion.

### Differential Diagnosis for the Noncontrast Head CT Findings

- ▶ Neoplasm
- ▶ Cerebritis

### Teaching Points

- ▶ The noncontrast head CT is used to identify hemorrhage.
- ▶ Little to no FLAIR MRI signal abnormality suggests that a stroke is <6 hours old.
- ▶ Diffusion-weighted MRI demonstrates increased signal within 30 minutes of symptom onset, providing the gold standard for detecting acute ischemia. A DWI abnormality larger than 70 cc is a contraindication for intra-arterial recanalization procedures at some institutions.
- ▶ Perfusion maps used to detect ischemic but viable tissue at risk of infarction (normal on DWI but abnormal on perfusion) are typically mean transit time, time-to-peak, time to maximum of the deconvolved residue function, and/or cerebral blood flow maps. Patients without at perfusion-diffusion mismatch are less likely to benefit from reperfusion therapy.

### Management

- ▶ Emergent head CT to exclude hemorrhage and hypodensity in more than one-third of the middle cerebral artery territory,
- ▶ Intravenous thrombolytic therapy for appropriate patients presenting within 4.5 hours of symptom onset.
- ▶ Intra-arterial recanalization procedures for appropriate patients with proximal vessel occlusions presenting within 6 hours of symptom onset.
- ▶ Supportive therapy including heparinization strict blood pressure control for patients who cannot receive other therapies.

## History

▸ 23-year-old postpartum female with headache and visual disturbance.

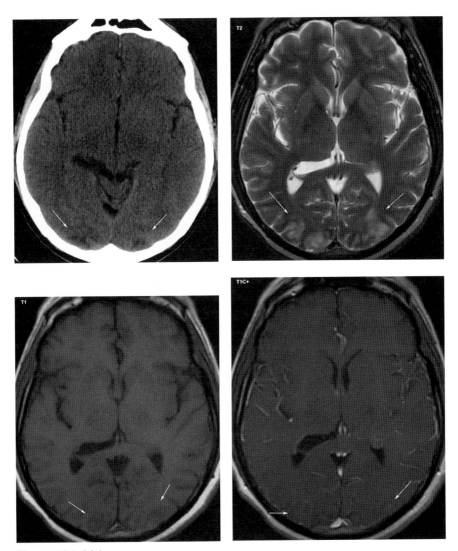

**Figures 96.1–96.4**

# Case 96   Posterior Reversible Encephalopathy Syndrome

## Findings

### Distribution

▶ Most common: Posterior circulation predilection involving the posterior temporal, parietal, and occipital lobes
▶ Less common: Frontal lobes (frequently in a border zone distribution), basal ganglia, and brainstem

### CT

▶ Patchy bilateral hypodense foci involving gray and subcortical white matter
▶ Hemorrhage in 20%
▶ +/- patchy enhancement

### MRI

▶ T1: Hypointense cortical/subcortical lesions
▶ T2 and FLAIR: Hyperintense cortical/subcortical lesions
▶ T1C+: Variable patchy enhancement
▶ T2*: Blooming if hemorrhage present
▶ DWI: Usually elevated (consistent with vasogenic edema) but can occasionally show restricted diffusion

## Differential Diagnosis

▶ Hypoglycemia
▶ Acute ischemia
▶ Status epilepticus
▶ Venous sinus thrombosis
▶ Infectious and inflammatory leukoencephalidites

## Teaching Points

▶ Neurologic disorder characterized by particular radiographic findings combined with clinical manifestations of headache, mental status change, seizure, and/or visual disturbances
▶ Associated with diverse conditions including
  ▪ Preeclampsia
  ▪ Acute/subacute hypertension
  ▪ Drug toxicity (chemotherapy agents)
  ▪ Autoimmune disorders
  ▪ Sepsis
▶ Pathogenesis
  ▪ Hypertension often common component
  ▪ Vasogenic edema (two leading theories)

1. Hypertension exceeds the limits of autoregulation, leading to breakthrough brain edema
2. Hypertension leads to cerebral autoregulatory vasoconstriction, ischemia, and subsequent brain edema

  ▪ Posterior circulation more susceptible to disturbances in autoregulation because of sparse sympathetic innervation
  ▪ Overlap with reversible cerebral vasoconstrictive syndrome in some patients

## Management

▶ Usually reversible if treated promptly
▶ Correct underlying conditions (e.g., treat hypertension, deliver child in preeclampsia)

## History

► 30-year-old female with protein S deficiency presents with headaches.

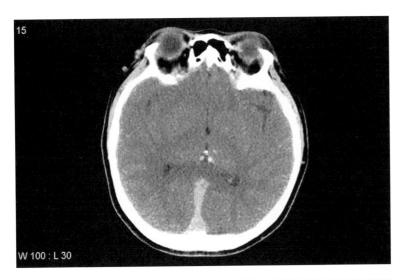

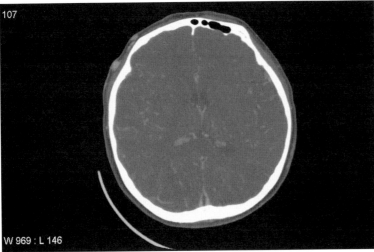

**Figures 97.1–97.2**

# Case 97   Acute Venus Sinus Thrombosis

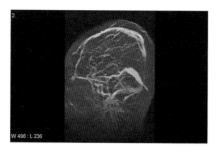
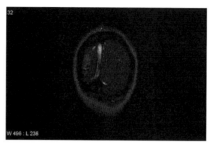
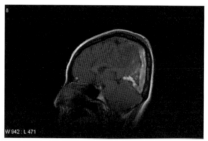

**Figures 97.3–97.5**

## Findings

▶ Noncontrast CT: in 20% of cases, direct visualization of hyperdense clotted venous sinus or cerebral vein; hypodensity and gyral swelling in nonarterial distribution; bilateral cerebral manifestations in cases of midline venous clot (e.g., bilateral thalamic involvement with deep venous clot or bilateral parasagittal involvement with superior sagittal sinus thrombus).

▶ CT venography: filling defect within the intracranial venous system; 95% sensitive.

▶ MRI: two-dimensional time-of-flight MR venography demonstrates absence of flow-related enhancement in clotted segment; susceptibility-weighted images also sensitive for cerebral venous clot.

## Differential Diagnosis

▶ Normal venous variants; pacchionian arachnoid granulations, insufficient CT scan delay resulting in poor opacification of venous system (recommend delay of 45 seconds after 3 cc/s bolus injection for CTV), polycythemia.

## Teaching Points

▶ Etiology: intracranial and systemic infections, immobilization, hypercoagulable disorders, malignancy, dehydration, pregnancy, oral contraceptives.

▶ Presentation: Unlike arterial infarcts, typically slower and more progressive onset of symptoms, which include headache, nausea/vomiting, papilledema, difficulty with vision, focal neurologic deficits, and seizures.

▶ Complications: edema, infarction, superimposed hemorrhage, hydrocephalus.

▶ Other pearls:

  ▪ Think of venous thrombosis in younger or middle age patients with severe headache or patients with stroke-like symptoms in absence of typical risk factors.

  ▪ Poor prognostic indicators: hemorrhage, involvement of deep venous system, and superimposed infection.

  ▪ Location in order of decreasing frequency: superior sagittal sinus, transverse sinus, straight sinus, cortical veins, deep venous system.

## Management

▶ Systemic anticoagulation with occasional direct transcatheter thrombolysis. Angioplasty with venous stenting performed anecdotally in cases of severe intracranial hypertension without clear long-term benefit.

## History

▶ 30-year-old male patient with persistent postural headache.

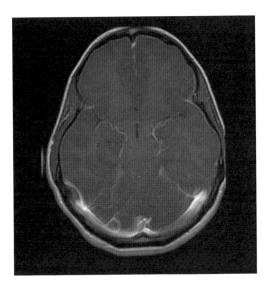 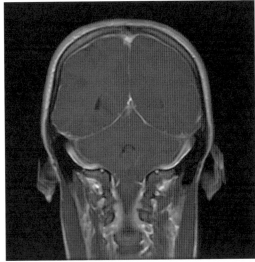

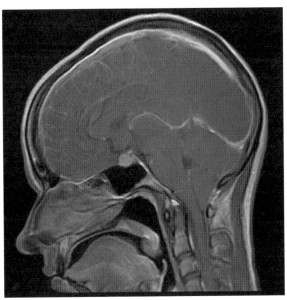

**Figures 98.1–98.3**

# Case 98  Intracranial Hypotension

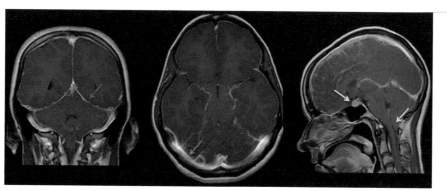

**Figure 98.4**

## Findings

### MRI

► Diffuse pachymeningeal enhancement (blue arrow) and prominence of dural venous sinuses (green arrow).

► Engorgement and prominence of the pituitary gland (yellow arrow).

► Bilateral subdural collections, cerebellar tonsillar descent, or herniation (light green arrow).

► Spinal imaging often shows prominence of the spinal epidural venous plexus and subdural/epidural collections.

## Differential Diagnosis

► Chiari 1 malformation

► Chronic meningitis

## Teaching Points

► Clinical presentation: Clinical syndrome characterized by a persistent postural headache, often with nausea and vomiting but also associated with a variety of focal neurologic findings.

► Etiology: Intracranial hypotension can be primary (spontaneous) or secondary to prior surgical procedures or trauma.

## Management

► Symptomatic management of headache initially. For persistent symptoms, identification of a CSF leak is important for a targeted epidural patch.

Further Readings

Chiapparini L, Ciceri E, Nappini S, et al. Headache and intracranial hypotension: neuroradiological findings. *Neurol Sci.* 25(3):s138–s141.

Forghani R, Farb RI. Diagnosis and temporal evolution of signs of intracranial hypotension on MRI of the brain. *Neuroradiology.* 50(12):1025–1034.

Rahman M, Sharatchandra S, Bidari R, Quisling G, Friedman WA. Spontaneous intracranial hypotension: dilemmas in diagnosis. *Neurosurgery.* 69(1):4–14– discussion 14.

## History

▸ 37-year-old female with history of asthma.

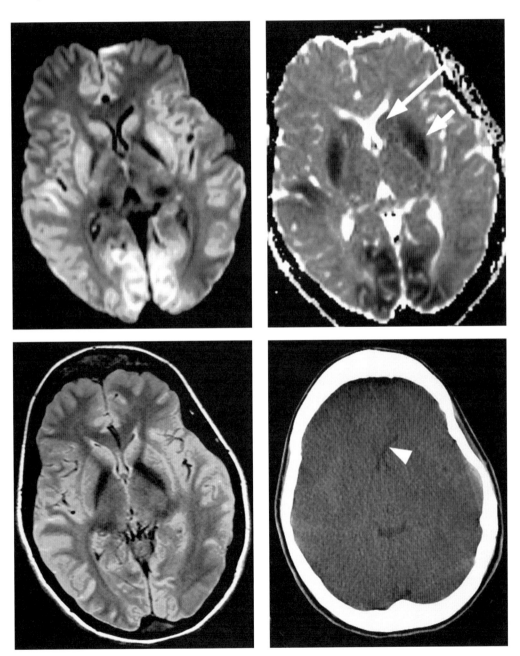

**Figures 99.1–99.4**

# Case 99   Hypoxic Ischemic Injury

## Findings

### MRI (Figure 99.2)

▶ Findings of acute hypoxic-ischemic injury (HII) to the brain
▶ Restricted diffusion involving areas of cortex and deep gray matter, with corresponding abnormally elevated T2 hyperintensity
▶ Areas of early abnormality reflect intrinsically elevated metabolic activity
▶ Deep gray matter nuclei; the caudate and putamen are indicated by long and short arrows, respectively, on the ADC image
▶ Occipital cortex
▶ More diffuse T2 hyperintensity involving gray and white matter and mild effacement of sulci, consistent with mild cerebral edema
▶ Relative sparing of frontal lobe gray and white matter

### CT (Figure 99.4)

▶ Diffuse loss of gray and white matter differentiation throughout the cerebrum, consistent with evolution of diffuse hypoxic-ischemic brain injury
▶ Marked effacement of the ventricles (arrowhead shows frontal horn of left lateral ventricle) and sulci as well as diffuse hypodensity throughout the cerebrum, consistent with diffuse cerebral edema

## Clinical Presentation

▶ HII may result from hypoperfusion, as with cardiac arrest; hypoxia, as with asphyxiation; or a combination of these
▶ Patterns of brain injury are markedly different in neonates, children, and adults, reflecting differences in brain maturity

## Pathophysiology

▶ HII results from a combination of hypoxia; decreased energy-rich metabolites (e.g., glucose, ketones, and fatty acids); and increased metabolic waste products (e.g., lactate)
▶ Acute hypoxia without ischemia, as with asphyxiation, is less injurious to the brain
▶ Certain brain tissues demonstrate selective vulnerability to HII, particularly gray matter including hippocampi, primary somatic motor and sensory, and deep gray matter nuclei

## Teaching Points

▶ Imaging findings of HII are extremely variable and depend on the age of the patient, the mechanism of injury, the imaging modality, and time since the HII event
▶ The pattern of brain injury reflects the mechanisms of injury and the selective vulnerability of brain structures

## Management

▶ MRI is much more sensitive than CT for evaluation of HII
▶ Imaging findings of hypoxic-ischemic injury may not be apparent immediately, and early imaging may appear normal
▶ Best prognostic data may be obtained from MRI approximately 72 hours after HII event
▶ Hypothermia may be used to decrease brain injury

# Section 2    Head, Neck, and Spine

## History

► None

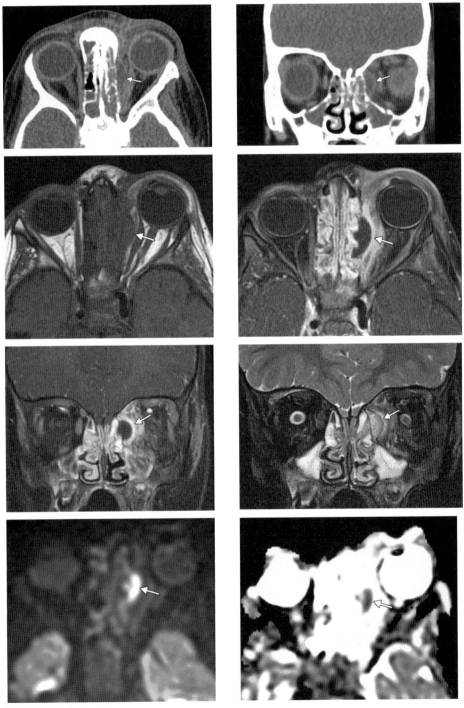

**Figures 100.1–100.8**

# Case 100  Orbital Subperiosteal Abscess

## Findings

▶ Axial (Figure 100.1) and coronal (Figure 100.2) contrast-enhanced CT images show an extraconal lenticular-shaped fluid collection (arrows) with rim-enhancement along the medial aspect of the left orbit resulting in proptosis. Stranding of the medial left orbital fat and eyelid are also present, indicative of orbital cellulitis. In addition, there is opacification of the ethmoid sinuses, left greater than right, consistent with sinusitis.

▶ Axial T1 (Figure 100.3), axial (Figure 100.4), and coronal (Figure 100.5) postcontrast fat-suppressed T1, and fat-suppressed coronal T2 (Figure 100.6) MRIs also show the rim-enhancing superiosteal abscess in the medial left orbit (arrows). The preseptal and postseptal cellulitis are more conspicuous on MRI than the corresponding CT. The linear low signal intensity stricture surrounding the fluid collection noted on the coronal T2 image represents the displaced periosteum. The diffusion-weighted image (Figure 100.7) and corresponding ADC map (Figure 100.8) show restricted diffusion within the abscess (arrows).

## Differential Diagnosis

▶ Subperiostealphlegmon
▶ Orbital abscess/cellulitis
▶ Subperiosteal hematoma
▶ Sinonasal or nasolacrimal duct mucocele
▶ Epidermoid
▶ Rarely, neoplasms, such as metastasis

## Teaching Points

▶ Orbital subperiosteal abscess most commonly results from ethmoid sinusitis.
▶ An elongated extraconal collection adjacent to lamina papyracea with peripheral enhancement is the typical appearance of subperiosteal abscess on CT and MRI. Restricted diffusion can be observed in the collection.
▶ Complications include orbital cellulitis, optic neuritis, retinal ischemia, superior ophthalmic vein and cavernous sinus thrombosis, meningitis, and intracranial abscess.

## Management

▶ CT with contrast is considered to be the first-line imaging modality for evaluating acute orbital infections.
▶ MRI with contrast is more sensitive than contrast-enhanced CT, particularly for delineating intracranial complications. Dedicated orbital protocol T2 and postcontrast T1 sequences are particularly helpful. In addition, postcontrast T1 sequences of the entire brain should also be performed.
▶ Intravenous antibiotics may be adequate treatment for small uncomplicated abscesses, especially in patients <10 years of age.
▶ Medial subperiosteal abscesses that fail medical therapy are usually drained endoscopically, whereas more extensive abscesses may require external drainage.

## History

► None

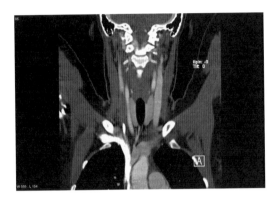 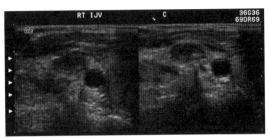

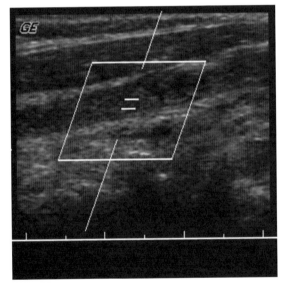

**Figures 101.1–101.3**

# Case 101   Internal Jugular Venous Thrombosis (IJVT)

## Findings

### Ultrasound

▶ Noncompressible vessel with mixed echogenicity intraluminal thrombus
▶ Absent flow on pulsed-wave Doppler

### CTA/MRA

▶ Intraluminal filling defect without enhancement
▶ Increased vessel diameter (acute thrombosis)
  ▪ In chronic thrombosis, the vessel may be smaller or unidentifiable
▶ ± edema or stranding of the perivascular fat (acute)
▶ Regional venous collaterals
  ▪ More common in chronic thrombosis

## Differential Diagnosis

▶ Tumor thrombus (e.g., sarcoma)
  ▪ Intraluminal filling may enhance

## Teaching Points

▶ Etiology
  ▪ Primary (10%): idiopathic thrombosis and thrombosis secondary to thoracic outlet syndrome
  ▪ Secondary (90%): central venous catheters; cancer (most commonly lung cancer and lymphoma/leukemia); coagulation abnormalities (antiphospholipid antibody, factor V Leiden mutation, prothrombin mutation); cervical infections (Lemierre syndrome); trauma; postsurgical complication
▶ Presentation: pain and induration over the affected side, cervical edema, arm edema, superficial venous collaterals
▶ Complications
  ▪ Pulmonary embolism: up to 10% of patients
  ▪ Postthrombotic syndrome: up to 15% of patients
  ▪ Intracranial propagation of the thrombus
  ▪ Rare: elevated intracranial pressures have been reported with bilateral acute IJVT

## Management

▶ Depends on the clinical setting and patient risk factors
▶ Treatment options include
  ▪ Systemic anticoagulation
  ▪ Line removal if catheter-associated thrombosis
  ▪ Superior vena cava filter placement
  ▪ Percutaneous interventions, such as mechanical thromebectomy or thromboaspiration (rarely necessary)
▶ Monitoring with Serial duplex ultrasound

## Further Reading

Gbaguidi X, Janvresse A, Benichou J, Cailleux N, Levesque H, Marie I. Internal jugular vein thrombosis: outcome and risk factors. *QJM*. 2011;104(3):209–219.

## History

▶ 21-year-old female who had a sore throat and respiratory distress.

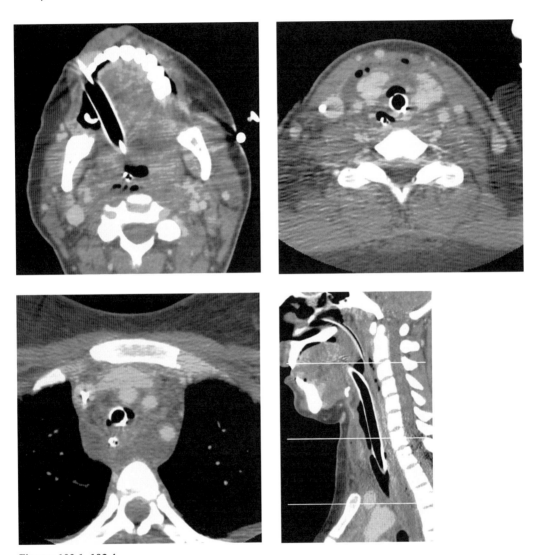

**Figures 102.1–102.4**

# Case 102  Prevertebral Abscess

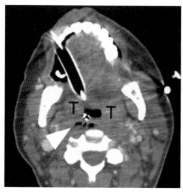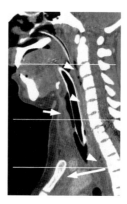

**Figures 102.5–102.6**

## Findings

- Findings of tonsillarphlegmon and prevertebral abscess extending into the mediastinum, resulting in descending necrotizing mediastinitis
- Air and fluid reflecting abscess in the prevertebral/retropharyngeal space (arrowheads), consistent with prevertebral abscess
- Increased prevertebral density that would be evident on neck radiographs and CT
- Air and fluid reflecting abscess in the visceral space anteriorly (short arrow)
- Air and fluid reflecting abscess in the mediastinum (long arrow), consistent with mediastinitis
- Phlegmon involving the palatine tonsils reflecting suppurative lymphadenitis (T)
- Extensive effacement of fat planes soft tissues of the neck reflecting infection and inflammation

## Differential Diagnosis: Cervical Prevertebral/Retropharyngeal Space Collection

- Infection: typically bacterial (streptococcus, staphylococcus)
- Inflammation: calcific tendonitis of the longuscolli
- Trauma: may result in prevertebral soft tissue swelling, edema, or hematoma
- Origin of infection
  - Head and neck, odontogenic, respiratory tract, salivary glands, pharynx, esophagus, cellulitis

## Pathophysiology

- The prevertebral space is a potential space that can be pathologically expanded
- Abscess in the prevertebral space can extend contiguously into the mediastinum, allowing for rapid progression of infection, and hence this is termed the "danger space"

## Clinical Presentation

- Infection typically extends into the prevertebral space, and so most patients have a history of recent infection in an adjacent space in the head and neck, such as the oral cavity, pharynx, or cervical spine
- Infection may progress rapidly after it enters the prevertebral space

## Teaching Points

- Prevertebral abscess is a rare and life-threatening complication that may result in descending necrotizing mediastinitis, associated with even higher mortality
- Danger space: potential space extending through the retropharyngeal space and mediastinum from the skull base to the diaphragm

## Management

- Prevertebral abscess has high mortality and warrants urgent intervention
- Empiric antibiotic coverage should be initiated immediately
- Surgical incision and drainage is indicated for significant collections
- Endotracheal intubation or tracheostomy may be required for respiratory distress

## History

▶ Pain, disability after cervical trauma ± radiculopathy, myelopathy.

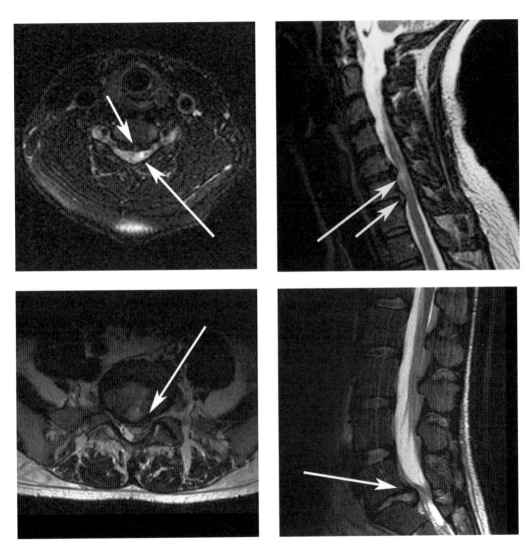

**Figures 103.1–103.4**

# Case 103  Acute Disk Herniation

## Findings

- ▶ Disk herniation with evidence of spinal trauma on imaging or history
- ▶ Morphology: Same appearance as degenerative disk herniation
- ▶ Radiography is insensitive for disk pathology
  - ▪ May see focal disk space narrowing
  - ▪ Focal kyphosis, traumatic spondylolisthesis, dislocated facet joints
  - ▪ Fracture or compression deformity
- ▶ CT findings
  - ▪ Soft tissue density in anterior or anterolateral epidural space; narrowing of disk space is a variable finding
  - ▪ Spinal fracture, facet subluxation
- ▶ MRI findings (best seen on T2WI)
  - ▪ Disk material effacing ventral CSF ± cord or nerve root compression
  - ▪ Cord edema may be present with cord compression
  - ▪ Possible disruption of posterior longitudinal ligament
  - ▪ Paraspinal effusion or hematoma

## Differential Diagnosis

- ▶ Nontraumatic disk herniation
- ▶ Epidural abscess, phlegmon
- ▶ Epidural tumor
- ▶ Epidural extension of vertebral metastases, aggressive hemangioma, lymphoma

## Teaching Points

- ▶ MRI is the modality of choice to evaluate intervertebral disks and the soft tissue contents of spinal canal
- ▶ Cervical region most common, followed by thoracic; lumbar region least common
- ▶ MRI of spine should be performed before reduction of facet dislocation

## Management

- ▶ Cord compression from traumatic herniation is a reported complication of reduction of cervical facet dislocation without discectomy
- ▶ Conservative management with surgery for those with persistent symptoms including weakness, sensory loss, and radiculopathy
- ▶ Percutaneous nucleoplasty can be used in patients who fail conservative management and are unwilling to undergo a more invasive technique, such as spinal surgery

## Further Readings

Dai L, Jia L. Central cord injury complicating acute cervical disc herniation in trauma. *Spine*. 20001;25(3):331–335, discussion 336.

Khashaba A. Acute intraosseous disc herniation. *Injury*. 2000;31(4):271–272.

Kreichati GE, Kassab FN, Kharrat KE. Herniated intervertebral disc associated with a lumbar spine dislocation as a cause of cauda equina syndrome: a case report. *Eur Spine J*. 2006;15(6):1015–1018.

Reddy AS, Loh S, Cutts J, Rachlin J, Hirsch JA. New approach to the management of acute disc herniation. *Pain Physician*. 2005;8(4):385–390.

Rizzolo SJ, Piazza MR, Cotler JM, Balderston RA, Schaefer D, Flanders A. Intervertebral disc injury complicating cervical spine trauma. *Spine*. 1991;16(6 suppl):S187–S189.

**History**

▶ Fever and acute or subacute spinal pain and tenderness

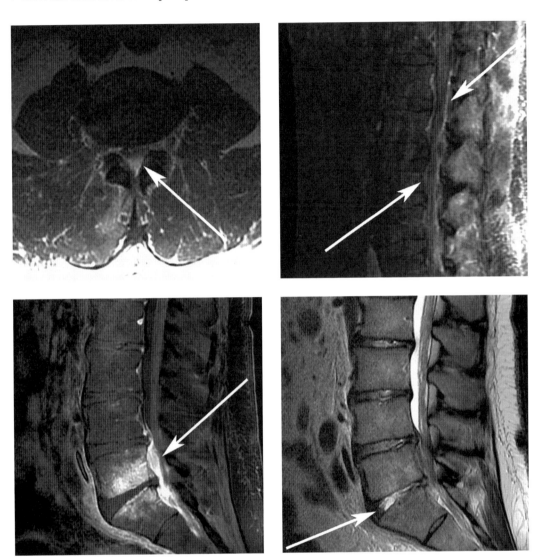

**Figures 104.1–104.4**

# Case 104  Epidural Abscess

## Findings

- ▶ CT Findings: Increased epidural soft tissue; may be difficult to distinguish from disk in ventral epidural space
- ▶ CECT: Enhancing epidural mass/collection narrowing the spinal canal
- ▶ MRI Findings
  - ■ T1WI: Isointense to hypointense to cord
  - ■ T2WI: Hyperintense
    - ■ Signal alteration in spinal cord secondary to compression, ischemia, or direct infection
  - ■ DWI: Typically restrict diffusion similar to abscess in brain.
  - ■ CE T1WI
    - ■ Homogeneously or heterogeneously enhancing phlegmon
    - ■ Peripherally enhancing necrotic abscess
    - ■ Diffuse dural enhancement in extensive abscess
    - ■ Enhancing prominent anterior epidural veins or basivertebral venous plexus adjacent to abscess
    - ■ Signal alteration in spinal cord secondary to compression, ischemia, or direct infection

## Differential Diagnosis

- ▶ Extradural metastasis
- ▶ Spinal epidural lymphoma
- ▶ Epidural hematoma
- ▶ Extruded/migrated disk
- ▶ Epidural lipomatosis

## Teaching Points

- ▶ Best imaging tool: sagittal and axial T2WI and T1WI MRI with gadolinium
- ▶ Epidural soft tissue with homogeneous or peripheral enhancement and adjacent spondylodiskitis characteristic of spinal epidural abscess
- ▶ Carefully assess cord for signs of signal changes
  - ■ Best seen on STIR and confirmed on axial T2WI
  - ■ DWI imaging useful to confirm cord extension of abscess

## Management

- ▶ Early empiric antibiotics with broad-spectrum coverage until causative pathogen isolated
- ▶ Emergent surgical decompression with abscess drainage advocated by some, even in absence of initial neurologic compromise
  - ■ This is because of the possibility of rapid progression of neurologic deficits despite appropriate medical therapy
- ▶ Medical therapy alone if substantial operative risks, extensive cranial-caudal involvement of spinal canal, or paralysis >48–72 hours
- ▶ Location (dorsal versus ventral) spinal epidural abscess plays role in determining treatment plan

## Further Readings

Tompkins M, Panuncialman I, Lucas P, Palumbo M. Spinal epidural abscess. *J Emerg Med*. 2010;39(3):384–390.
Zimmerer SME, Conen A, Müller AA, Sailer M, Taub E, Flückiger U, et al. Spinal epidural abscess: aetiology, predisponent factors and clinical outcomes in a 4-year prospective study. *Eur Spine J*. 2011;20(12):2228–2234.

## History

▶ Back pain and tenderness ± fever.

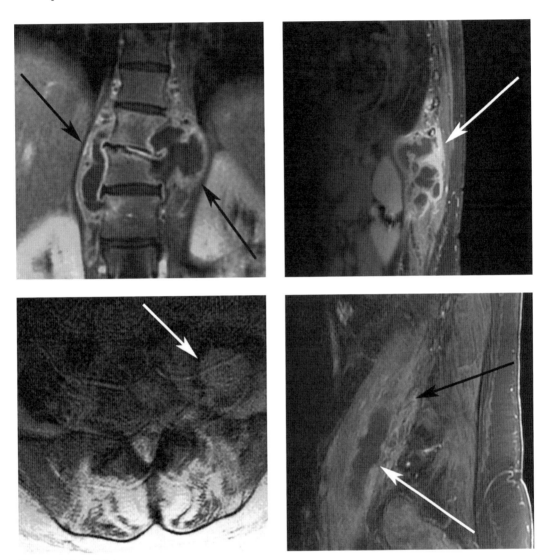

**Figures 105.1–105.4**

# Case 105  Paraspinal Abscess

## Findings

- Paravertebral enhancing phlegmon or peripherally enhancing liquified collection
- May extend into the psoas, iliacus, or posterior paraspinous muscles (erector spinae)
- Can be solitary, multiple, and/or multiloculated
- Extend along subligamentous and muscles planes
- Obliterated soft tissue fascial planes
- Intraspinal epidural extension with cord compression
- Involvement of lateral epidural space with neuroforaminal narrowing
- Radiography: Nonspecific findings
  - Osseous abnormalities present in delayed fashion (see diskitis/osteomyelitis findings)
  - May identify an enlarged psoas shadow or a paraspinal soft tissue density
- CT finding: Poorly defined soft tissue density with low-density intramuscular collection
- CECT
  - Diffuse or peripheral enhancement
  - Enhancing disk space
- MRI findings
  - T1WI
    - Isointense to hypointense
    - May be difficult to distinguish from normal musculature
    - Obscuration of musculofascial planes
  - T2WI
    - Hyperintense fluid collection and surrounding muscle
    - Hypointense rim
  - DWI
    - Evidence of restricted diffusion increases conspicuity of epidural, vertebral, and paraspinal abscesses
  - T1WI C+
    - Phlegmon: Diffuse enhancement
    - Abscess: Peripherally enhancing fluid collections
- Best imaging tool: Sagittal and axial T1WI C+ and T2WI MRI

## Differential Diagnosis

- Neoplasm, primary or metastatic
- Desmoid, calcifications with low signal intensity
- Retroperitoneal hematoma
- Extramedullary hematopoiesis

## Teaching Points

- Evaluate adjacent vertebral bodies and intervertebral disk spaces for spondylodiskitis
- Well-defined paraspinal collections with thin and smooth abscess wall along with presence of paraspinal or intraspinal abscess and thoracic spine involvement are more suggestive of tuberculous versus pyogenic spondylitis

## Management

- Intravenous antibiotics
- Analgesic medications
- Percutaneous catheter drainage
- Surgical debridement
- Spinal stabilization in some cases

## History

▶ Severe, localized back pain ± radiculopathy.

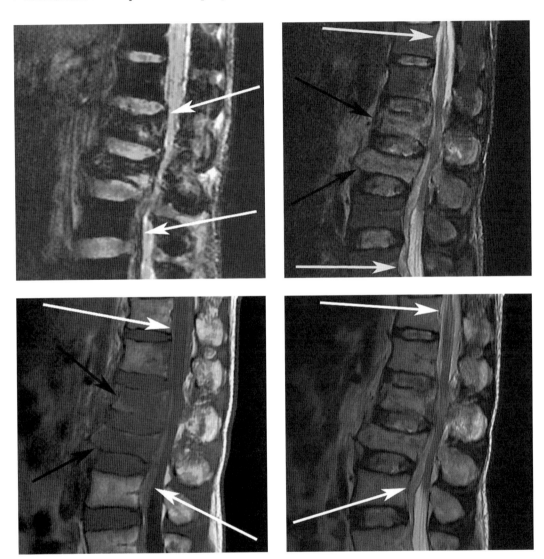

**Figures 106.1–106.4**

# Case 106  Epidural Hematoma

## Findings

- ▶ Best diagnostic clue: fusiform, extradural mass-like process with signal characteristics of hemorrhage on MRI
- ▶ May be located at any level of spine
  - ▪ Most commonly seen in the dorsal epidural space extending over multiple levels
- ▶ CT: Hyperdense, extradural collection
- ▶ MRI findings
  - ▪ T1WI
    - ▪ Epidural fluid collection, signal depends on age of hematoma
    - ▪ Acute hemorrhage can be similar in signal to cord or CSF on T1WI
    - ▪ Subacute (methemoglobin) is hyperintense to CSF and cord
  - ▪ T2WI: Epidural fluid collection, signal depends on age of hematoma
- ▶ STIR: Hyperintense relative to cord and epidural fat
- ▶ T2* GRE: Accentuates susceptibility artifact from blood products
- ▶ T1WI C+: Mild peripheral enhancement may be seen with subacute hematoma

## Differential Diagnosis

- ▶ Epidural abscess (or phlegmon)
- ▶ Epidural lipomatosis
- ▶ Epidural tumor
- ▶ Extramedullary hematopoiesis
- ▶ Ossification of posterior longitudinal ligament
- ▶ Sequestered disk fragment

## Teaching Points

- ▶ When spontaneous, considered a neurosurgical emergency
- ▶ MRI study of choice; include contrast injection and fat saturation
- ▶ Active extravasation may enhance
- ▶ CT may help identify hemorrhage when MRI confusing

## Management

- ▶ Surgical evacuation/decompression may be necessary to alleviate compression of spinal cord or cauda equina syndrome
- ▶ If no significant neurologic compromise, may be managed conservatively
- ▶ Vitamin K injection or fresh frozen plasma to reverse coagulopathies

### Further Readings

Al-Mutair A, Bednar D. Spinal epidural hematoma. *J Am Acad Orthop Surg.* 2010;18:494–502.
Sklar EML, Donovan Post JM, Falcone S. MRI of acute spinal epidural hematomas. *J Comput Assist Tomogr.* 1999;23(2):238.
Zhong W, Chen H, You C, Li J, Liu Y, Huang S. Spontaneous spinal epidural hematoma. *J Clin Neurosci.* 2011;18(11):1490–1494.

## History

► None

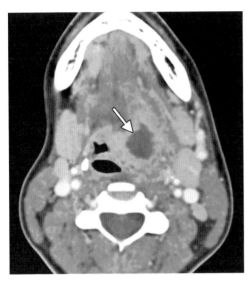 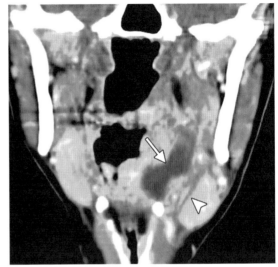

**Figures 107.1–107.2**

# Case 107 Peritonsillar Abscess

## Findings

▶ Axial (Figure 107.1) and coronal (Figure 107.2) CT images show a low-attenuation collection with surrounding enhancement located in the left lingual tonsil and extending into the parapharyngeal space. The linear low-attenuation structure that traverses the left submandibular gland likely represents a thrombosed glandular vein (arrowhead).

## Differential Diagnosis

▶ Phlegmon
▶ Suppurative lymphadenopathy
▶ Squamous cell carcinoma
▶ Benign mixed tumor
▶ Tonsillar hypertrophy

## Teaching Points

▶ Peritonsillar abscess can result as a complication of tonsillitis and consists of a collection of pus situated external to the tonsillar capsule, tonsillar fossa, and superior constrictor muscle, extending into the parapharyngeal space and beyond.
▶ Findings on CT can include enlargement and enhancement of the tonsil and a fluid collection with rim enhancement.
▶ Patients with peritonsillar abscess may present with sore throat, dysphagia, fever, and trismus.
▶ Extension of peritonsillar abscess posterolaterally into the carotid sheath can lead to jugular vein thrombosis and carotid artery pseudoaneurysm.
▶ Hounsfield unit measurement has not been found to be reliable in distinguishing abscess from phlegmon.

## Management

▶ Peritonsillar abscess is generally diagnosed clinically and treated with antibiotics and drainage.
▶ CT and MRI have high sensitivity for detecting abscess formation and its precise location and extension of disease.
▶ Needle aspiration or intraoral ultrasound can also be performed to confirm the diagnosis.
▶ Associated complications should be sought on imaging, especially in cases that do not respond to initial treatment.

Further Readings

Gonzalez-Beicos A, Nunez D. Imaging of acute head and neck infections. *Radiol Clin North Am.* 2012;50(1):73–83. doi: 10.1016/j.rcl.2011.08.004.

Smith JL 2nd, Hsu JM, Chang J. Predicting deep neck space abscess using computed tomography. *Am J Otolaryngol.* 2006;27(4):244–247.

Johnson RF, Stewart MG. The contemporary approach to diagnosis and management of peritonsillar abscess. *Curr Opin Otolaryngol Head Neck Surg.* 2005;13:157–160.

## History

▸ None

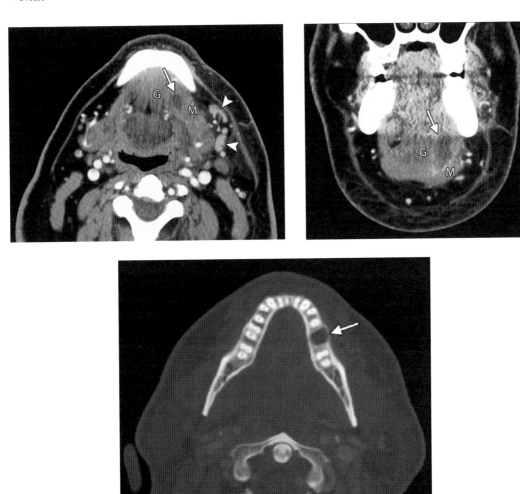

**Figures 108.1–108.3**

# Case 108  Sublingual Abscess

### Findings

▶ Axial (Figure 108.1) and coronal (Figure 108.2) contrast-enhanced CT images show a fluid collection with ill-defined peripheral enhancement (arrows) in the left sublingual space, splaying apart the adjacent genioglossus-geniohyoid complex (G) and mylohyoid (M) muscles. Asymmetrically enlarged reactive left level IB lymph nodes are present (arrowheads). There is also thickening of the left platysma and stranding of the surrounding subcutaneous fat.

▶ Axial CT image (Figure 108.3) in the bone window shows a recent tooth extraction cavity (arrow).

### Differential Diagnosis

▶ Phlegmon/cellulitis without abscess
▶ Neoplasm: squamous cell carcinoma, salivary gland tumor
▶ Ranula
▶ Dermoid/epidermoid

### Teaching Points

▶ The sublingual space lies within the floor of the mouth; contains the sublingual gland, submandibular duct, and lingual neurovascular bundle; and is bounded by the mylohyoid inferolaterally, the genioglossus and geniohyoid medially, and intrinsic tongue muscles superiorly.

▶ Sublingual abscess most commonly results from dental disease and submandibular or sublingual duct stenosis.

▶ Thickening of the ipsilateral plastysma, stranding of the subcutaneous fat, and regional lymphadenopathy may be present as secondary signs of infection on contrast-enhanced CT.

▶ Sublingual abscess may not display peripheral enhancement in the very early stages.

▶ Ludwig angina is a rapidly progressive cellulitis of the bilateral sublingual spaces that can extend into the submandibular space and as far as the mediastinum. This condition can result in dangerous airway compromise.

### Management

▶ Antibiotic and surgical drainage.
▶ Emergent intubation if there is associated Ludwig angina.
▶ The role of imaging is to confirm the diagnosis, delineate the extent of disease, and identify associated complications.

### Further Readings

La'porte SJ, Juttla JK, Lingam RK. Imaging the floor of the mouth and the sublingual space. *RadioGraphics.* 2011;31(5):1215–1230.

Jason A. McKellop, Suresh K, Mukherji MD, Emergency Head and Neck Radiology: Neck Infections. *Appl Radiol.* Volume 39, Number 7, July-August 2010; http://appliedradiology.com/Issues/2010/07/Articles/AR_07-08-10_Mukherji/Emergency-Head-and-Neck-Radiology-Neck-Infections.aspx

## History

▶ Fever and severe back pain

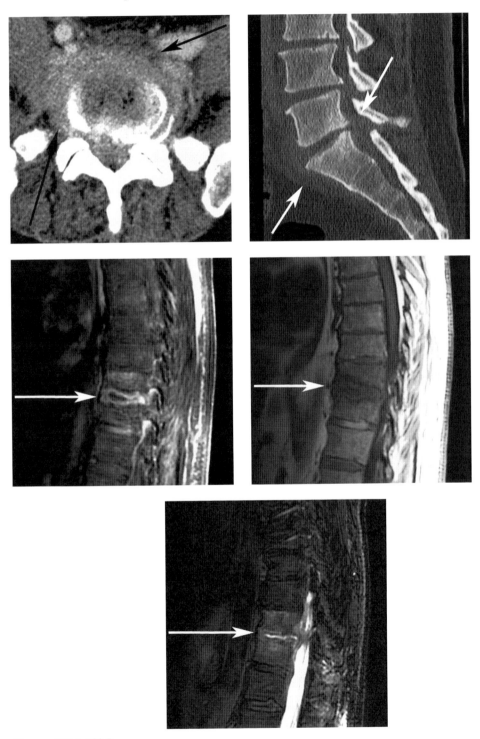

**Figures 109.1–109.5**

# Case 109  Pyogenic Diskitis Osteomyelitis

## Findings

- Disk space narrowing, end plate destruction, bone marrow edema
- Most common in lumbar spine; almost always in vertebral body (95%) with sparing of posterior elements
- Soft tissue changes around spine
- Radiographic findings normal in early disease and/or nonspecific, (i.e., focal end plate destruction)
- Disk space "air" related to vacuum phenomenon, excludes infection
- CT better displays focal end plate destructive changes, specificity added with fluid in disk space and stranding/fluid in paraspinal soft tissues
  - ± paraspinal abscess
- MRI findings
  - Abnormally enhancing fluid in the disk space with associated vertebral end plate signal changes and bone marrow edema
    - Bone marrow edema can often be best seen on T1W images
    - STIR or T2 with FS can also increase sensitivity
  - Paraspinal edema and phlegmon helps to distinguish from neoplasm
  - May see enhancement in psoas muscle, paraspinal soft tissues, or epidural space
  - Enhancement within disk space may be subtle, T1 FS and multiplanar imaging postcontrast helpful

## Differential Diagnosis

- Amyloid deposition disease
- Mechanical disk disease/neuropathic spine (may enhance)
- Neoplasms extending across disk spaces (multiple myeloma, lymphoma, metastatic disease)
- Inflammatory arthritis and crystal deposition

## Teaching Points

- Radiographs may be nonspecific or appear normal in early disease
- MRI is most sensitive and specific

## Management

- Antimicrobial therapy is mainstay of treatment
- Surgical debridement typically not indicated
- Surgical stabilization if significant instability
- Rarely percutaneous drainage of psoas abscess

## Further Readings

DeSanto J, Ross JS. Spine infection/inflammation. *Radiol Clin North Am.* 2011;49(1):105–127.

Dunbar JAT, Sandoe JAT, Rao AS, Crimmins DW, Baig W, Rankine JJ. The MRI appearances of early vertebral osteomyelitis and discitis. *Clin Radiol.* 2010;65(12):974–981.

Tali ET. Spinal infections. *Eur J Radiol.* 2004 May;50(2):120–33.

**History**

▸ Sudden onset paralysis.

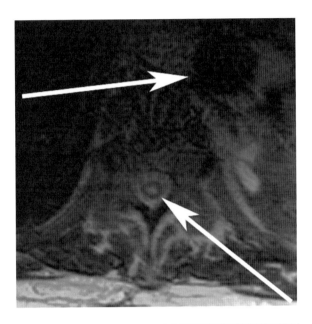

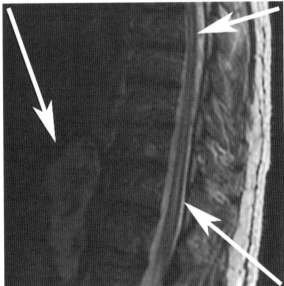

**Figures 110.1–110.2**

# Case 110  Spinal Cord Infarction

## Findings

### General Features

▶ Best diagnostic clue: Central "owl's eye" pattern; hyperintensity on T2WI within cord
▶ Location: Distal half of thoracic cord → arterial border zone
▶ Size: Usually more than one vertebral body segment
▶ Morphology: Central hyperintensity on T2WI, which involves central gray matter, more variable involvement of cord periphery

### CT Findings

▶ NECT: Noncontributory
▶ CTA
  ▪ Useful to define underlying aortic disease causing infarct, or to discover other etiologies mimicking cord infarct (arteriovenous dural fistula)
  ▪ Not directly useful for identifying ASA because lack of visualization of ASA does not prove diagnosis

### MRI Findings

▶ T1WI
  ▪ Slight cord expansion in acute phase
  ▪ Cord atrophy as chronic finding
  ▪ Hemorrhage conversion → hyperintense (rare)
▶ T2WI
  ▪ Hyperintense central gray matter or entire cross-sectional area
▶ DWI
  ▪ Hyperintense, as in brain infarcts
▶ MRA
  ▪ Dynamic contrast enhanced
▶ Assess other etiologies that may mimic infarct, such as dural arteriovenous fistula
▶ Not directly useful for identifying ASA because lack of visualization of ASA does not prove diagnosis

### Imaging Recommendations

▶ Best imaging tool: MRI with contrast and diffusion DWI

## Differential Diagnosis

▶ Multiple sclerosis
▶ ADEM/viral myelitis
▶ Neuromyelitis optica
▶ Spinal arteriovenous dural fistula
▶ Radiation myelopathy
▶ Cord infection

## Teaching Points

▶ Look for associated vertebral body infarctions as confirmatory evidence of cord ischemia in aortic disease
▶ Classic imaging appearance: T2 hyperintensity involving anterior horn cells

## Management

▶ Anticoagulation with heparin and aspirin
▶ Steroids
▶ Supportive care and rehabilitative physical therapy

## History

▸ None

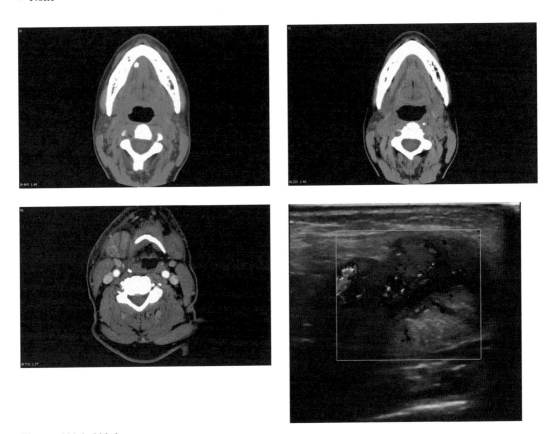

**Figures 111.1–111.4**

# Case 111  Submandibular Sialadenitis

## Findings

### Acute

- ▶ Ipsilateral enlargement of the submandibular gland, often painful
- ▶ Dilation of the submandibular duct (Wharton duct) secondary to ductal stenosis or obstructing calculus
- ▶ Often associated cellulitis and myositis
- ▶ Most commonly *Staphylococcus aureus* infection

### Chronic

- ▶ Ipsilateral atrophy of the submandibular gland, often painless
- ▶ Dilation of submandibular duct secondary to chronic calculi and salivary stasis

### Secondary Sialedenitis

- ▶ Typically a result of ductal obstruction secondary to squamous cell carcinoma in the floor of the mouth

## Differential Diagnosis

- ▶ Dental infection
- ▶ Squamous cell carcinoma nodal metastases
- ▶ Benign mixed tumor
- ▶ Submandibular gland carcinoma

## Teaching Points

- ▶ Best imaging tool is contrast-enhanced CT
- ▶ If no calculi visualized on study, consider other etiology, such as Sjögren syndrome; Kuttner tumor; or sialadenosis secondary to diabetes, hypothyroidism, cirrhosis

## Management

- ▶ Hydration, compression and massage, and antibiotics for infected gland
- ▶ Consider gland excision in recurrent cases
- ▶ Incision and drainage of abscess if present

## Further Readings

Avrahami E, et al. CT of submandibular gland sialolithiasis. *Neuroradiology*. 1996;38(3):287–290.

Capps EF, et al. Emergency Imaging Assessment of Acute, Nontraumatic Conditions of the Head and Neck. *Radiographics*. 2010;30:1335–1352.

## History

▶ Patient with a neoplastic process with motor weakness and sensory complaints.

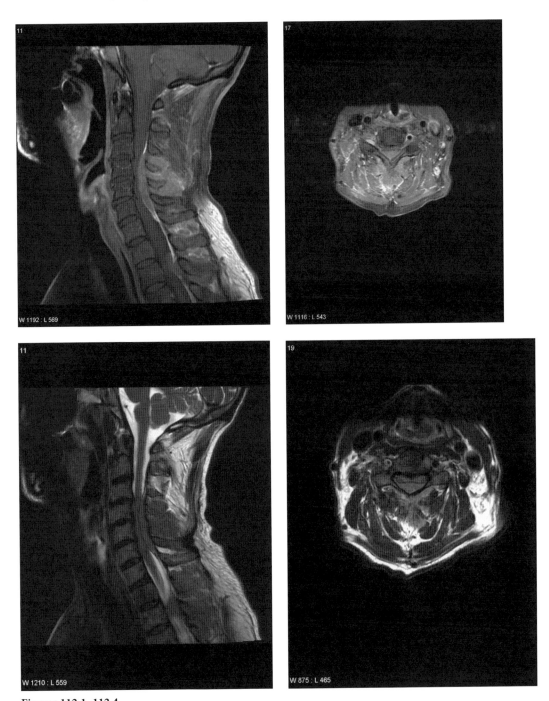

**Figures 112.1–112.4**

# Case 112  Cord Compression

## Findings

### MRI

▶ Axial and sagittal images of the cervical spine, demonstrating an enhancing mass indenting the spinal cord
▶ Cord compression can be graded by anteroposterior cord diameter: if anteroposterior cord diameter is greater than two-thirds the cord diameter at the C1 spinal level it is defined as mild, if is less than two-thirds the cord diameter at the C1 level it is defined as severe.

## Differential Diagnosis

▶ Myelitis (inflammatory, infectious)
▶ Cord infarction

## Teaching Points

▶ Cord compression from neoplasm can occur in multiple areas. More than one-third of patients have tumor at multiple sites, thus the whole spine should be imaged.
▶ MRI is the best examination to delineate the spinal cord.
▶ CT can assist in surgical planning. Allows characterization of osseous disease and osseous anatomy. Does not allow full characterization of the spinal cord.
▶ Myelography: Contrast allows the outer contour of the cord to be visualized, cord swelling can be seen. Can be used in patients with contraindications to MRI.

## Management

▶ Corticosteroids, surgical decompression, radiotherapy

## Further Readings

Cook AM, Lu TN, Tomlinson MJ, Vaidya M, Wakeley CJ, Goddard P. Magnetic resonance imaging of the whole spine in suspected malignant spinal cord compression: impact on management. *Clin Oncol.* 1998;10:39–43 (doi: 10.1016/S0936-6555(98)80111-8).

Husband DJ, Grant KA, Romaniuk CS. MRI in the diagnosis and treatment of suspected malignant spinal cord compression. *Br J Radiol.* 2001;74:51–23 (doi:10.1148/rg.304095706).

# Section 3    Chest

## History

▸ 41-year-old female on recently initiated chemotherapy in respiratory distress admitted to ICU.

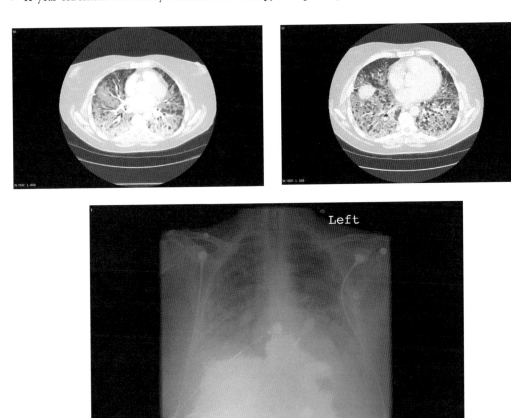

**Figures 113.1–113.3**

# Case 113 Diffuse Alveolar Damage

## Findings

▸ CXR shows hazy opacity greatest in the mid to lower lung zones
▸ Axial CT images demonstrate scattered and diffuse areas of ground-glass opacity

## Differential Diagnosis

▸ Multifocal pneumonia
▸ Pulmonary edema
▸ Pulmonary hemorrhage
▸ Toxic inhalation
▸ ARDS

## Teaching points

▸ Nonspecific appearance of lungs with scattered and/or diffuse areas of ground-glass opacity
▸ Initially is scattered pattern of opacity but becomes more confluent and diffuse; chronic diffuse alveolar damage results in pulmonary fibrosis
▸ Fibrosis can start to develop in weeks but more easily detected on CT

## Management

▸ Most commonly, expectant management and removal of insult (i.e., stop offending drug)

### Further Readings

Rossi SE, Erasmus JJ, McAdams HP, Sporn TA, Goodman PC. Pulmonary drug toxicity: radiologic and pathologic manifestations. *RadioGraphics.* 2000;20(5):1245–1259.

Bydash J, Kasmani R, Naraharisetty K. Metal fume-induced diffuse alveolar damage. *J Thorac Imaging.* 2010 May;25(2):W27–W29.

## History

▸ 28-year-old patient with no history of cardiac disease presenting with shortness of breath after aggressive fluid resuscitation.

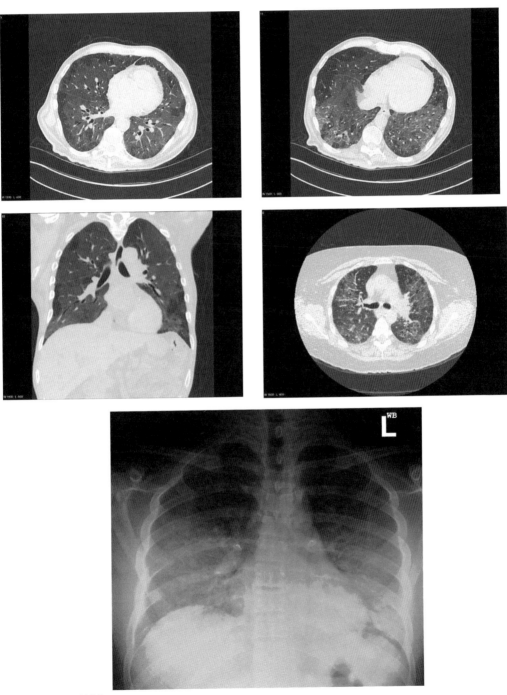

**Figures 114.1–114.5**

# Case 114  Pulmonary Edema, Noncardiogenic

## Findings

▶ Nonspecific hazy opacity greatest on chest radiograph throughout lungs
▶ Axial CT images demonstrate diffuse areas of ground-glass opacity

## Differential Diagnosis

▶ Pulmonary edema
▶ Pulmonary hemorrhage
▶ Toxic inhalation
▶ Diffuse alveolar damage
▶ ARDS
▶ Multifocal pneumonia

## Teaching points

▶ Unlike cardiogenic pulmonary edema, in noncardiogenic edema, there is typically no evidence of cardiomegaly, apical vascular redistribution, Kerley lines
▶ Alveolar opacities and diffuse ground-glass opacities on CT
▶ Noncardiogenic pulmonary edema is caused by changes in permeability of pulmonary small vessels
▶ Multiple causes of noncardiogenic pulmonary edema include drowning, fluid overload, inhalational injury, neurogenic pulmonary edema, allergic reaction, ARDS

## Management

▶ Most commonly, expectant management and removal of insult
▶ ICU admission if severe respiratory distress with mechanical ventilation

### Further Readings

Gluecker T, Capasso P, Schnyder P, et al. Clinical and radiologic features of pulmonary edema. *RadioGraphics*. 1999;19:1507–1531.

Milne EN, Pistolesi M, Miniati M, et al. The radiologic distinction of cardiogenic and noncardiogenic edema. *AJR Am J Roentgenol*. 1985;144(5):879–894.

## History

▶ 45-year-old female with a fever and cough.

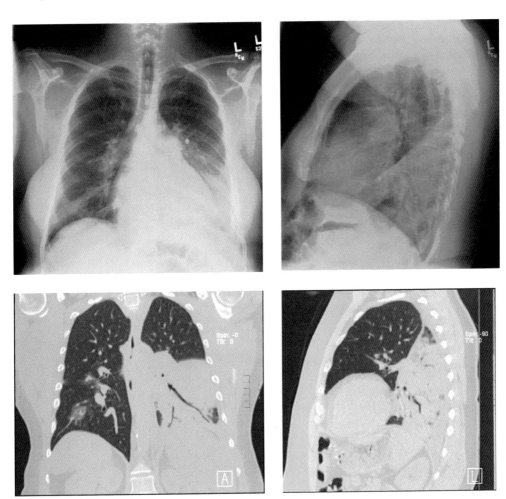

**Figures 115.1–115.4**

# Case 115  Pneumonia

## Findings

▶ Frontal (Figure 115.1) and lateral (Figure 115.2) radiographs of the chest demonstrate dense opacity occupying the left lower lobe. Note the well-demarcated left major fissure .

▶ The left heart border is well demonstrated but there is obscuration of the left hemidiaphragm, consistent with a lower lobar process. This is called the silhouette sign.

▶ There is increased opacity over the lower vertebral bodies compared with the upper vertebral bodies. This is called the spine sign.

▶ There are air bronchograms .

▶ These findings are consistent with lobar pneumonia, which was confirmed by chest CT. Coronal (Figure 115.3) and sagittal (Figure 115.4) reformatted images are shown. There are additional foci of infection seen in the right lung on CT.

## Differential Diagnosis

▶ Edema
▶ Hemorrhage
▶ Atelectasis or lobar collapse
▶ Aspiration
▶ Bronchoalveolar carcinoma
▶ Cryptogenic organizing pneumonia/eosinophilic pneumonia

## Teaching Points

▶ Pneumonia is a common diagnosis, which is classified based on its anatomic location within the lung.

▶ Lobar pneumonia occurs when infectious organisms reach the subpleural zone of the lung. This results in alveolar damage, hemorrhage, and rapid proliferation of the organism, which can spread to the adjacent lung through the pores of Kohn. Lobar pneumonia is much less common because of improved antibiotic treatment.

▶ The most common cause of community-acquired pneumonia is *S. pneumoniae*. Other causes of lobar pneumonia include *Klebsiella*, Legionella pneumophila, and *Mycoplasma pneumoniae*.

▶ Radiographic signs of pneumonia include
  ▪ Air bronchograms: branching linear or tubular lucencies representing bronchi or bronchioles passing through opacified parenchyma (Figure 115.3 and 115.4)
  ▪ Silhouette sign: obliteration of the borders of the heart, mediastinum, or diaphragms secondary to opacified adjacent lung parenchyma
  ▪ Spine sign: increasing opacity over the vertebral bodies of the lower thorax is indicative of a lower lobar process (Figure 115.2).
  ▪ Bulging fissure sign: the lobe appears expanded because of voluminous edema. This is classically seen with *Klebsiella*.

## Management

▶ Antibiotic treatment

## History

▶ None

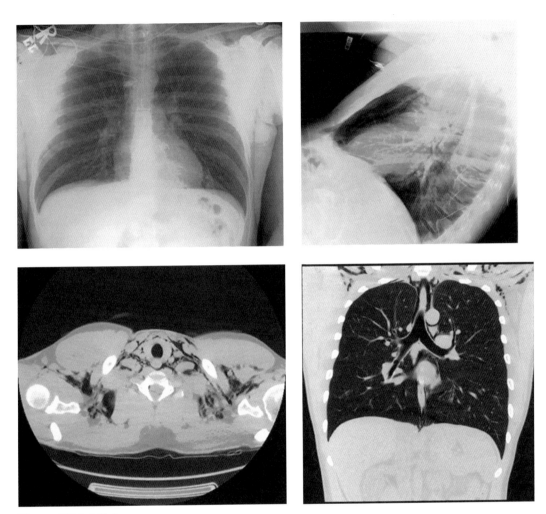

**Figures 116.1–116.4**

# Case 116  Pneumomediastinum

## Findings

▶ Subcutaneous emphysema: Air within the neck and thoracic soft tissues.

▶ Continuous diaphragm sign: A continuous band of air seen underneath the heart on a frontal view of the chest.

▶ Spinnaker sail sign: Elevation of the thymus by mediastinal air; seen in infants.

▶ Ring around the artery sign: Lucent air is seen surrounding the pulmonary artery or aorta. This finding is best appreciated on the lateral view.

## Differential Diagnosis

▶ Medial pneumothorax

▶ Pneumomediastinum

▶ Pneumopericardium

## Teaching Points

▶ Pneumomediastinum can be caused by intrathoracic or extrathoracic sources. Intrathoracic sources include alveolar rupture, esophageal rupture, or tracheal rupture Extrathoracic sources include dissecting air from the peritoneal cavity or the retroperitoneum. The most common source for mediastinal air with children and adults is alveolar rupture secondary to increased intrapulmonary pressure.

▶ Presentation of patients with pneumomediastinum is highly variable and may range from completely asymptomatic to excruciating chest pain. Classically on physical examination patients may present with a Hamman sign, which is a "crunching" sound heard in the precordium, which is synchronous with the heartbeat; this is usually present in about 50% of patients.

## Management

▶ Often no treatment is necessary because the body reabsorbs the mediastinal air. If pneumomediastinum is complicated by pneumothorax then a chest tube is placed.

## Further Readings

Zylak CM, Standen JR, Barnes GR, Zylak CJ. Pneumomediastinum revisited. *RadioGraphics*. 2000;20:1043–1057.
Bejvan SM, Godwin JD. Pneumomediastinum: old signs and new signs. *AJR Am J Roentgenol*. 1996;166:1041–1048.

## History

▶ 35-year-old female with dyspnea and leg pain.

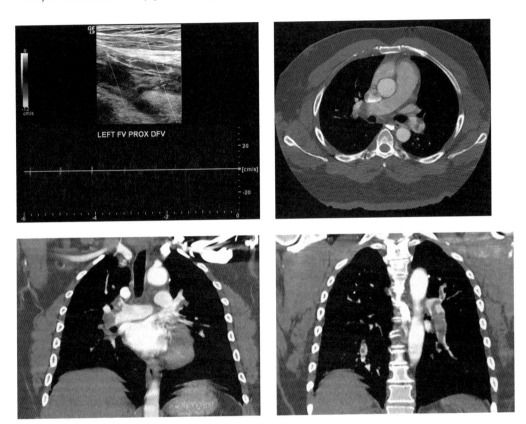

**Figures 117.1–117.4**

# Case 117 Pulmonary Embolism/Deep Vein Thrombosis

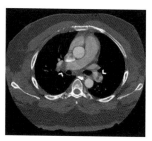 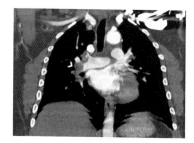 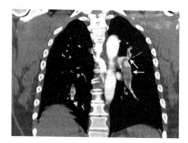

**Figures 117.5–117.7**

## Findings

▶ Figures 117.1: Ultrasonographic interrogation of the left femoral vein demonstrates echogenic filling defect devoid of color flow or venous wave form.
▶ Figures 117.3: Contrast-enhanced CT of chest demonstrates multiple filling defects in the distal main pulmonary arteries (arrows).
▶ Figures 117.5, 117.6 and 117.7: Coronal reformatted images of the same patient show multiple emboli (arrowhead) including saddle embolus in the upper and lower left pulmonary artery (arrows).

## Differential Diagnosis

▶ Acute pulmonary embolus
▶ Chronic pulmonary embolus

## Teaching Points

▶ Pulmonary embolism is occlusion of the pulmonary arterial tree secondary to emboli.
▶ Pulmonary embolism commonly results from deep vein thrombosis; however, it can also occur in the setting of embolization of air, fat, amniotic fluid, talc, or other foreign bodies.
▶ The emboli obstruct normal blood flow through the lungs and can increase the pressure in the pulmonary arterial tree and right ventricle.
▶ Extremity venous ultrasound findings include echogenic filling defects, lack of compression or augmentation, and absence of color flow on Doppler.
▶ Most chest radiographs are normal.
▶ Rarely, a peripheral, wedge-shaped opacity (Hampton hump) is noted. This finding represents a pulmonary infarct.
▶ Contrast-enhanced chest CT demonstrates filling defects in the pulmonary arterial tree.

## Management

▶ Anticoagulation
▶ Thrombolysis
▶ Thrombectomy

### Further Readings

Stein PD, Fowler SE, Goodman LR, et al. Multidetector computed tomography for acute pulmonary embolism. *N Engl J Med.* 2006;354(22):2317–2327.
Le Gal G, Righini M, Parent F, van Strijen M, Couturaud F. Diagnosis and management of subsegmental pulmonary embolism. *J Thromb Haemost.* 2006;4(4):724–731.
Schaefer-Prokop C, Prokop M. MDCT for the diagnosis of acute pulmonary embolism. *Eur Radiol.* 2006;15(suppl 4):D37–D41.

## History

▶ 49 year old with high fevers, right-sided chest pain, and dyspnea.

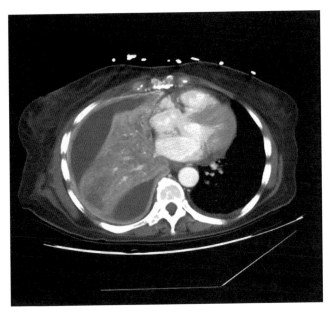

**Figure 118.1**

# Case 118  Empyema

## Findings

▶ Axial CT demonstrates a right-sided pleural effusion with rim enhancement representing the split pleura sign and underlying right lung pneumonia

## Differential Diagnosis

▶ Pleural effusion (exudative)
▶ Lung abscess
▶ Evolving hemothorax if in setting of trauma

## Teaching Points

▶ Clinical symptoms may be nonspecific including fever, elevated WBC, chest pain, shortness of breath
▶ CT typically demonstrates fluid density collection with possible locules of gas, septa, and a split pleura sign on contrast-enhanced studies given that the parietal and visceral layers are divided by the empyema
▶ Chest radiograph shows pleural effusion and potential loculated appearance of effusion
▶ Ultrasound can reveal nonsimple fluid in the pleural space, septations, or debris

## Management

▶ Prompt evacuation of the empyema with antibiotics
▶ Consider surgical (VATS) and/or chest tube placement
▶ Fibrinolytics can also be placed into pleural cavity to break up loculations and septations

### Further Readings

Desai H, Agrawal A. Pulmonary emergencies: pneumonia, acute respiratory distress syndrome, lung abscess, and empyema. *Med Clin North Am.* 2012;96(6):1127–1148.

Weldon E, Williams J. Pleural disease in the emergency department. *Emerg Med Clin North Am.* 2012;30(2):475–499.

## History

► 54-year-old male with chest pain.

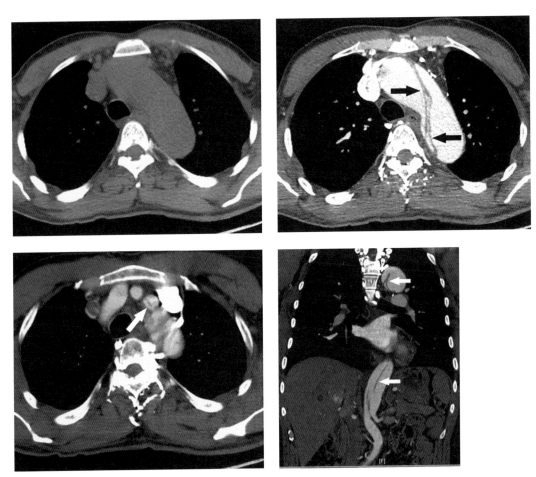

**Figures 119.1–119.4**

# Case 119  Aortic Dissection (Stanford Type A)

## Findings

### Chest Radiograph

▸ May be normal in up to 12.4% of patients with dissection
▸ The most common finding is a widened mediastinum (61.6%)

### CT

▸ Noncontrast images may show displaced intimal calcification. High attenuation within the aortic wall indicates the presence of intramural hematoma, which may clinically mimic or coexist with acute aortic dissection
▸ Anintimal flap separates the false and true lumens ( black and white arrows in axial and coronal images); the false lumen is usually larger than the true lumen
▸ Thin bands of low attenuation representing residual media may be seen in the false lumen; this is known as the cobweb sign.
▸ The beak sign refers to a wedge-shaped area of hematoma at the edge of the false lumen that creates a plane into which the false lumen can expand

### MRI

▸ An intimal flap is best seen on spin-echo "black blood" sequences
▸ A GRE cine sequence can be used to differentiate slow flow from thrombus within the false lumen, and can evaluate for aortic regurgitation if the dissection involves the aortic root

## Differential Diagnosis

▸ Intramural hematoma
▸ Tortuous aorta
▸ Thrombosed aortic aneurysm
▸ Traumatic aortic injury

## Teaching Points

▸ Stanford Type A dissection
  ▪ Intimal tear and/or associated intramural hematoma involves the ascending aorta, proximal to the origin of the left subclavian artery (60%–70% of cases, including the above case)
  ▪ Dissection flap may involve coronary arteries, and may also extend into the great vessels (arrow)
  ▪ Stanford Type A dissection may extend to involve the descending aorta (arrow)
  ▪ Mortality may result from rupture into the pericardial space resulting in cardiac tamponade
▸ Stanford Type B dissection
  ▪ Intimal tear involves the descending aorta, distal to the origin of the left subclavian artery and extending caudally
  ▪ Dissection flap may involve celiac, mesenteric, and renal arteries

## Management

▸ Type A dissection requires urgent surgical repair
▸ Type B dissection is managed medically unless the patient is unstable or there is evidence of vascular compromise to an organ

## History

▸ 72-year-old female with chest pain.

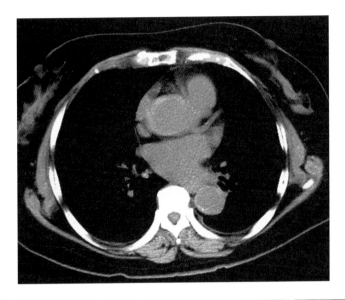

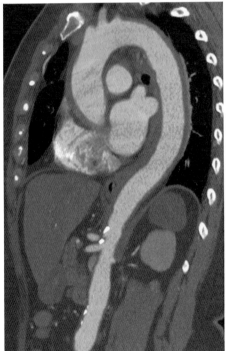
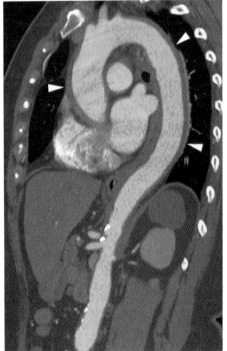

**Figures 120.1–120.3**

# Case 120 Aortic Intramural Hematoma

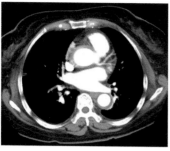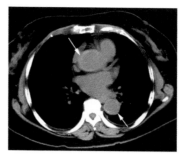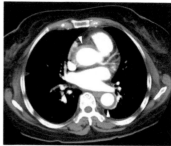

**Figures 120.4–120.6**

## Findings

### CT

▶ Noncontrast images show high-density hematoma within the wall of the thoracic and/or abdominal aorta (arrows) and may also show displaced intimal calcification

▶ Contrast-enhanced images make diagnosis difficult because the nonenhancing intramural hematoma may appear similar to luminal thrombus (arrowheads)

### MRI

▶ Can be used to help diagnose or determine age of intramural hematoma

▶ Acute intramural hematoma is hyperintense on "white-blood" images and isointense on "black-blood" images

▶ Cine phase-contrast or GRE sequences can be used to differentiate from communicating aortic dissection

## Differential Diagnosis

▶ Classic or thrombosed aortic dissection

▶ Hematoma associated with penetrating atherosclerotic ulcer

▶ Atheroma or intraluminal thrombus

▶ Aortitis

▶ Retroperitoneal fibrosis or lymphoma

## Teaching Points

▶ Classic intramural hematoma results from spontaneous hemorrhage of the vasa vasorum within the media, usually caused by hypertension

▶ CT, including noncontrast imaging, is the modality of choice

▶ Classified in same manner as aortic dissection

　■ Stanford Type A intramural hematoma involves the ascending aorta, beginning proximal to the origin of the left subclavian artery, and may extend caudally

　■ Stanford Type B intramural hematoma involves the descending aorta, beginning distal to the origin of the left subclavian artery

　■ Associated conditions and complications

　■ May coexist with penetrating ulcer or classic dissection

　■ May lead to dissection or aneurysm caused by weakening of the aortic wall

　■ Associated penetrating atherosclerotic ulcer or ulcerlike projection indicates increased risk of future complications

　■ Ulcerating lesions should be distinguished from focal intramural contrast enhancement or intramural blood pools, which do not clearly communicate with the true lumen and are of unlikely clinical significance

　■ Patients not treated surgically should receive imaging follow-up

## Management

▶ Usually treated in the same fashion as aortic dissection

　■ Type A requires urgent surgical repair

　■ Type B is managed medically unless the patient is unstable or there is evidence of vascular compromise to an organ

## History

▸ 75-year-old female with acute shortness of breath.

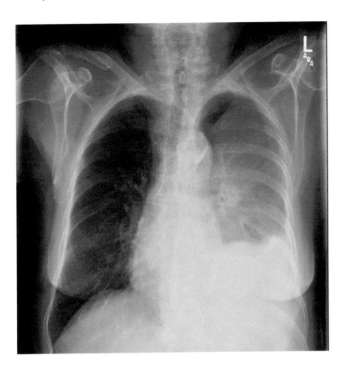

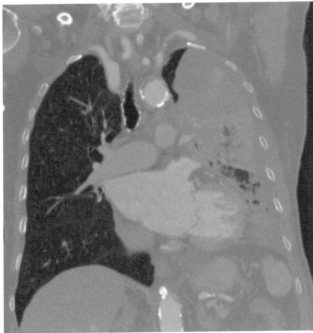

**Figures 121.1–121.2**

# Case 121  Lobar Collapse

## Findings

- Frontal chest radiograph (Figure 121.1) and coronal reformat from a subsequent chest CT (Figure 121.2) demonstrate veil-like opacity in the left middle and upper lung zones
- There is crescentic lucency adjacent to the aortic arch
- There is elevation of the left hilum, indicative of volume loss in the left upper lobe
- There is a speculated mass in the left hilum and a left pleural effusion

## Differential Diagnosis

- Airway obstruction secondary to bronchogenic carcinoma, endobronchial secretions, or endobronchial tumors, such as carcinoid
- Malpositioned endotracheal tube
- Airway compression secondary to fluid, mass, or lymphadenopathy
- Scarring

## Teaching Points

- Radiographic findings of lobar collapse include veil-like opacities; opacities with sharp borders; and shifting of the mediastinal contents, hilum, and fissures toward the region of suspected volume loss.
- Luftsichel ("air sickle") sign, as seen in this case, is most commonly a manifestation of left upper lobe collapse with wedging of the aerated superior segment of the left lower lobe between the collapsed lung and the aorta creating a periaortic lucency.
- In left upper lobe collapse, the upper lobe collapses anteriorly and superiorly against the chest wall with resultant hyperexpansion of the left lower lobe, which often tents the left hemidiaphragm.
- Another notable radiographic sign of lobar collapse is the "reverse S sign of Golden" in which the right minor fissure is displaced superiorly and assumes a convex inferior border medially and a concave inferior border laterally secondary to collapse of the right upper lobe.

## Management

- Cross-sectional imaging with CT should be performed to assess for obstructing lesions
- Bronchoscopy may be performed to remove the offending lesion

### Further Readings

Blankenbaker DG. The luftsichel sign. *Radiology*. 1998;208(2):319–320.
Gupta P. The Golden S sign. *Radiology*. 2004;233(3):790–791.
Lubert M, Krause GR. Patterns of lobar collapse as observed radiographically. *Radiology*. 1951;56(2):165–182.

## History

▶ 25-year-old patient recently rescued by firefighters from inhalation of smoke from burning house.

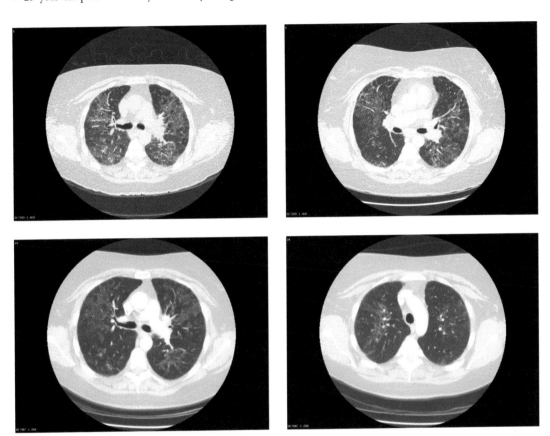

**Figures 122.1–122.4**

# Case 122   Toxic Inhalation

### Findings

▸ Axial CT images demonstrate diffuse ground-glass opacity

### Differential Diagnosis

▸ Multifocal pneumonia
▸ Pulmonary edema
▸ Pulmonary hemorrhage
▸ Diffuse alveolar damage
▸ ARDS
▸ PCP if signs of infection

### Teaching Points

▸ Nonspecific appearance of lungs, diffuse and scattered areas of ground-glass opacity
▸ Tree-in-bud opacities may also be present given inflammatory process also involving small airways

### Management

▸ Most commonly, expectant management and oxygen
▸ Laryngoscopy and bronchoscopy may be necessary to assess complications of airway
▸ Treat other concurrent comorbidities, such as burns, depending on inhalation injury

### Further Readings

Rossi SE, Erasmus JJ, McAdams HP, Sporn TA, Goodman PC. Pulmonary drug toxicity: radiologic and pathologic manifestations. *RadioGraphics.* 2000;20(5):1245–1259.

Bydash J, Kasmani R, Naraharisetty K. Metal fume-induced diffuse alveolar damage. *J Thorac Imaging.* 2010 May;25(2):W27–W29.

## History

► Swelling of right upper extremity.

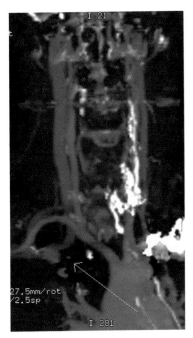

**Figure 123.1**

# Case 123   SVC Obstruction

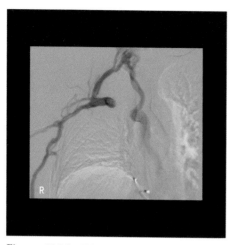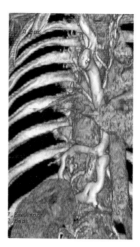

**Figures 123.2–123.3**

## Findings

▶ CT coronal reformat images demonstrating obstruction of the SVC (arrow)
▶ Venous angiography demonstrates filling of a dilated azygous vein through collaterals
▶ Three-dimensional reformat demonstrating filling of a dilated azygous vein through collaterals

## Differential Diagnosis

▶ Mediastinal mass
▶ Bronchogenic neoplasm
▶ Intravascular SVC thrombosis

## Teaching Points

▶ Often, history and physical examination yield diagnosis but imaging can confirm a mass obstructing the SVC
▶ Large mass can be seen on radiograph or CT in the region of the SVC
▶ Collateral circulation on contrast-enhanced CT can also be often visualized
▶ Obliteration or narrowing of SVC can be visualized on CT
▶ Obstruction caused by neoplastic invasion of the SVC and hemodynamically significant narrowing
▶ Intravascular thrombus may also be found in association
▶ Collateral circulation involving the azygous vein, hemiazygous vein, intercostal vein, and internal mammary veins can form
▶ Symptoms include dyspnea, arm swelling, chest pain, dysphagia, headache, nasal stuffiness, light headedness, and dramatic facial swelling in complete or near complete obstruction
▶ Early in clinical course, patient may be asymptomatic

## Management

▶ CT is more accurate than chest radiograph in providing accurate detailed anatomic evaluation for location and extent of neoplastic pathology obstructing SVC
▶ Stenting of SVC could be considered
▶ Chemotherapy or radiotherapy to treat primary tumor and lesion obstructing SVC
▶ Surgical management

## Further Readings

McCurdy MT, Shanholtz CB. Oncologic emergencies. *Crit Care Med.* 2012;40(7):2212–2222.
Lepper PM, Ott SR, Hoppe H, et al. Superior vena cava syndrome in thoracic malignancies. *Respir Care.* 2011;56(5):653–666.

# Section 4    Abdomen

## History

▶ 38-year-old male with fever, malaise, and jaundice.

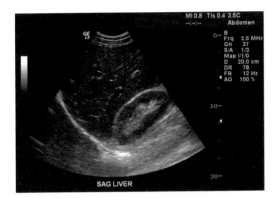 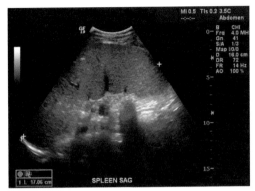

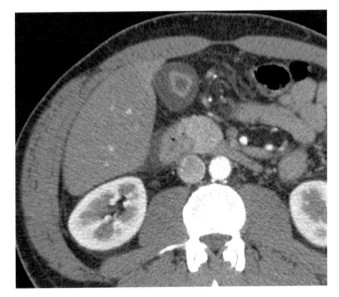

**Figures 124.1–124.3**

# Case 124  Hepatitis

## Findings

### Acute

- Diffuse hepatic edema, resulting in diffuse decrease in echogenicity or density of the liver; this may be particularly pronounced around the portal triads
- Hepatomegaly, splenomegaly, porta hepatis lymphadenopathy, and ascites
- Gallbladder wall thickening; often greater than with cholecystitis, and with a negative sonographic Murphy sign
- Heterogeneous enhancement on CT
- US
  - "Starry-sky" appearance of liver: caused by relative increased echogenicity of the portal triads against the diffusely hypoechoic liver parenchyma
  - Relative increased echogenicity of ligamentum venosum and falciform ligament
  - Hypoechoic liver echotexture becomes more similar to that of the spleen and renal cortex

### Chronic

- Diffuse heterogeneity and coarsening of liver echotexture or density; this is caused by a combination of regenerating nodules, steatosis, fibrosis, and necrosis
- Hepatic atrophy, with a retracted irregular capsule; especially of the right lobe, possibly with compensatory hypertrophy of the left and caudate lobes
- Loss of definition or silhouetting of the portal veins on ultrasound

## Differential Diagnosis

- Hepatic steatosis
- Hepatic congestion
- Diffuse lymphoma, hepatocellular carcinoma, or metastatic disease

## Teaching Points

- Viral hepatitis is the most common cause; other causes include alcohol, autoimmune, drug induced, radiation induced, and nonalcoholic steatohepatitis
- In severe fulminant cases, can be acutely fatal without liver transplant
- Chronic hepatitis increases the risk of developing hepatocellular carcinoma, especially if caused by hepatitis B virus

## Management

- Antiviral therapy
- Alcohol cessation
- Hepatitis B vaccine is available for prophylaxis
- Hepatitis B immune globulin for empiric treatment in cases of suspected acute exposure

## Further Readings

Dienstag JL. Hepatitis B virus infection. *N Engl J Med.* 2008;359:1486–1500.
Mortelé KJ, Segatto E, Ros PR. The infected liver: radiologic-pathologic correlation. *RadioGraphics.* 2004;24(4):937–955.
Abu-Judeh HH. The "starry sky" liver with right-sided heart failure. *AJR Am J Roentgenol.* 2002 Jan;178(1):78.

## History

▶ Right upper quadrant pain, nausea, and vomiting. Hemodynamically unstable with leukocytosis and high alkaline phosphatase.

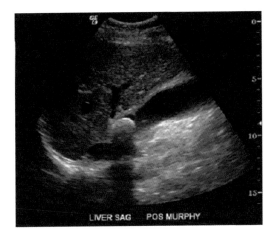
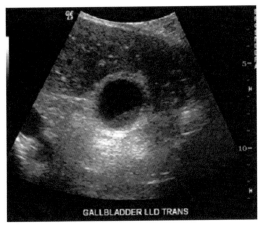
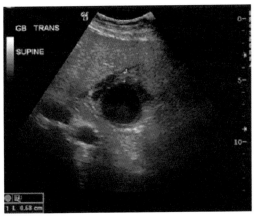

**Figures 125.1–125.3**

# Case 125  Acute Cholecystitis

## Findings

- Ultrasound image demonstrates a large gallstone at the gallbladder neck (Figure 125.1)
- Ultrasound image demonstrates gallbladder wall thickening (Figure 125.2)
- Ultrasound images demonstrate sludge within a gallbladder with thickened and edematous wall (Figures 125.3)

## Differential Diagnosis

- Gallbladder wall thickening from portal hypertension, ascites, and hypoalbuminemia

## Teaching Points

- Usual presentation is right upper quadrant pain, nausea, and/or vomiting.
- Occurs in about one-third of patients with gallstones.
- 95% caused by calculous obstruction in the gallbladder neck or cystic duct resulting in increased intraluminal pressure and distention and at times superimposed infection.
- Acalculous cholecystitis seen in patients with trauma, mechanical ventilation, hyperalimentation, postoperative state, diabetes mellitus, vascular insufficiency, prolonged fasting, burns, and postpartum state.
- Complications include gangrenous cholecystitis, emphysematous cholecystitis, gallbladder perforation, cholecystoenteric fistula, porcelain gallbladder resulting from chronic or recurrent cholecystitis, which in turn may result in gallbladder carcinoma.
- Ultrasound is modality of choice for evaluation of cholecystitis, both sensitive and specific.
- Ultrasound most sensitive findings: cholelithiasis and sonographic Murphy sign (maximal tenderness over the gallbladder as seen by ultrasound).
- Additional ultrasound findings: Gallbladder wall thickness >3 mm, gallbladder wall edema, pericholecystic fluid.

## Management

- Cholecystectomy, laparoscopic favored
- Percutaneous cholecystostomy catheter for the unstable patient

### Further Reading

Hanbidge A, Buckler P, O'Malley M, Wilson S. From the RSNA Refresher Courses: imaging evaluation for the acute pain in the right upper quadrant. *RadioGraphics*. 2004;24:1117–1135.

## History

▸ 89-year-old female with acute onset right upper abdominal pain.

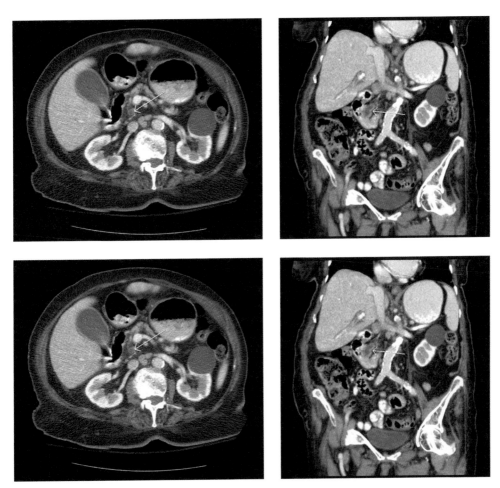

**Figures 126.1–126.4**

# Case 126 Acute Cholangitis

## Findings

- Coronal image from a contrast-enhanced CT of the abdomen demonstrates irregular dilatation of the distal common bile duct, which measured up to 10 mm in maximum dimension.
- Axial image from a contrast-enhanced CT of the abdomen demonstrates the "target sign": high-density material within the gallbladder (likely sludge) surrounded by low-density bile.

## Imaging Findings

### Ultrasound

- Dilatation, narrowing, or wall thickening of biliary ducts
- Echogenic material within the duct (pus)
- Stones (gallbladder or bile duct)

### CT

- Biliary ductal dilatation
- High-density material within the duct (pus)
- "Bull's eye": dense stone surrounding by low-density bile
- Look for hepatic abscesses (potential complication)

### MRCP

- Stones = low signal filling defects
- Bile = increased signal
- Structures, prestenotic biliary dilatation

### Fluoroscopy

- Irregular dilatation of bile ducts
- Stone = filling defect
- May see communication with hepatic abscesses

## Differential Diagnosis

- Primary sclerosing cholangitis (UC)
- AIDS-related recurrent cholangitis
- Chemotherapy cholangitis

## Teaching Points

- Ascending cholangitis: bacterial infection of intrahepatic and extrahepatic biliary system secondary to biliary obstruction
- Classic clinical presentation: Charcot triad (fever, right upper quadrant pain, jaundice)
  - Elevated WBC, bilirubin, alkaline phosphatase, positive blood cultures
  - Age 20–50 years
- Choledocholithiasis (number one cause); also, iatrogenic (post-ERCP)

## Management

- Antibiotics (for gram-negative bacteria)
- Intervention to remove stone or relieve stricture; 100% mortality if not decompressed!

## Further Readings

Statdx.com

Hanau LH, Steigbigel NH. Acute cholangitis. *Infect Dis Clin North Am*. 2000;14(3):521–546.

## History

▸ 46-year-old woman with intermittent abdominal pain especially after fatty meal.

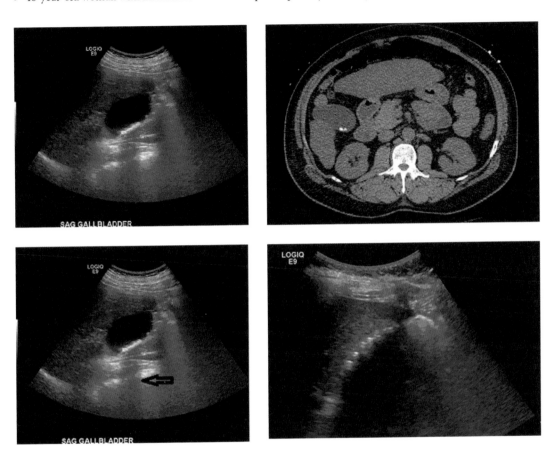

**Figures 127.1–127.4**

# Case 127 Gallstones/Cholelithiasis

## Findings

- ▶ Ultrasound image of the gallbladder demonstrating shadowing gallstones
- ▶ CT demonstrating hyperdense foci consistent with gallstones
- ▶ Black open arrow denotes posterior acoustic shadowing
- ▶ Wall echo shadow sign, resulting from multiple gallstones in a contracted gallbladder

## Differential Diagnosis

- ▶ Tumefactive sludge
- ▶ Cholesterol polyps
- ▶ Adenomyomatosis

## Teaching Points

- ▶ Approximately 25 million adults in the United States have cholelithisis, women more often than men.
- ▶ Prevalence increases with age.
- ▶ Because of supersaturation of bile constituents, usually cholesterol.
- ▶ Aggravated by high-fat diet, sedentary lifestyle, and genetic predisposition.
- ▶ Association with obesity, diabetes, oral contraceptives, ileal disease, total parenteral nutrition, cirrhosis, and spinal cord injury.
- ▶ Ultrasound characteristics of gallstones include hyperechoic structures within the gallbladder that are usually mobile with patient position. Gallstones usually demonstrate posterior acoustic shadowing.
- ▶ Wall echo shadow sign (Figure 127.4): anterior wall of the gallbladder is echogenic, below which is a thin, dark line of bile, and a highly echogenic line of superficial stones with associated posterior shadowing. Deeper stones are the posterior aspect of the gallbladder is not visible.
- ▶ CT findings include hyperdense structures within the gallbladder. They may have nitrogen gas inside the gallstones that may form the classic "Mercedes-Benz" sign.
- ▶ Complications include biliary colic, choledocholithiasis, acute cholecystitis, gallbladder perforation, pancreatitis, biliary fistula, Mirizzi syndrome, porcelain gallbladder, increasing risk of gallbladder carcinoma

## Management

- ▶ Cholecystectomy if symptomatic

## Further Reading

Bortoff G, Chen M, Ott D, Wolfman N, Routh W. Gallbladder stones: imaging and intervention. *RadioGraphics*. 2000;20:751–766.

## History

▶ Vomiting and epigastric pain.

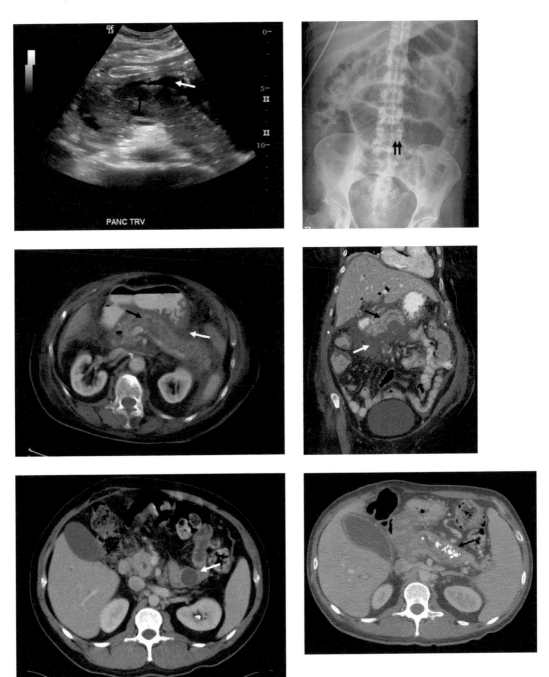

Figures 128.1–128.6

# Case 128  Acute Pancreatitis

### Findings

▶ Transverse ultrasound of the pancreas (Figure 128.1) demonstrates an enlarged and hypoechoic pancreas (black arrow), consistent with edema. There is peripancreatic fluid (white arrow), consistent with inflammation. These findings were confirmed on axial (Figure 128.3) and coronal reformat (Figure 128.4) images of the pancreas from a contrast-enhanced CT.

▶ Frontal radiograph of the abdomen (Figure 128.2) demonstrates several loops of dilated small bowel in the epigastrum (double black arrows), representative of ileus secondary to inflammation from the adjacent pancreatitis. This is the "sentinel loop sign."

### Differential Diagnosis

▶ Pancreatic carcinoma
▶ Lymphoma
▶ Metastatic disease
▶ Perforated duodenal ulcer

### Teaching Points

▶ Pancreatitis is largely a clinical diagnosis made in patients with fever, nausea, and epigastric pain who have elevated serum amylase and lipase. The role of imaging is primarily to assess the severity and complications of the disease.

▶ Alcohol, gall stones, infection, iatrogenia, hyperlipidemia, drugs, autoimmune disorders, and anatomic variability can all result in pancreatitis.

▶ Both ultrasound and CT demonstrate an enlarged, edematous pancreas with surrounding fluid, fat stranding, and possible abscesses (Figures 128.3, 128.4, and 128.5).

▶ Radiography may show dilated loops of small bowel (Figure 128.2, "the sentinel loop sign") from nearby pancreatic inflammation or the "colon cut off sign."

▶ Complications from pancreatitis include: necrosis, abscess formation, pseudoaneurysm formation, portosplenic vein thrombosis, shock, disseminated intravascular coagulation, and sepsis.

▶ Pseudocysts (Figure 128.5) and pancreatic calcifications (Figure 128.6) are pathognomonic for chronic pancreatitis.

### Management

▶ Keep the patient NPO to rest the pancreas
▶ Identify the cause of the pancreatitis

### Further Readings

Balthazar EJ. Acute pancreatitis: assessment of severity with clinical and CT evaluation. *Radiology.* 2002;223(3):603–613.
Balthazar EJ. Complications of acute pancreatitis: clinical and CT evaluation. *Radiol Clin North Am.* 2002;40(6):1211–1227.

## History

▸ 78-year-old woman on chemotherapy with abdominal pain.

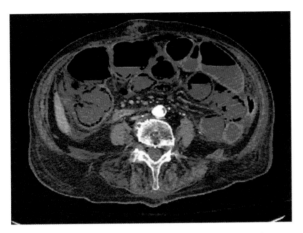

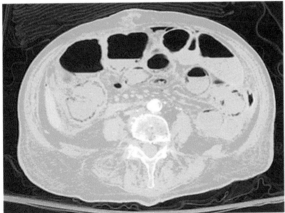

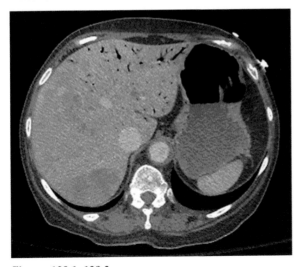

**Figures 129.1–129.3**

# Case 129  Pneumatosis Intestinalis

## Findings

- Linear and round foci of air within the intestinal wall
- Pneumatosis intestinalis is emphasized on lung windows
- Branching foci of air within the periphery of the liver denotes portal venous air in another patient

## Differential Diagnosis

None.

## Teaching Points

### Pathogenesis

- Gas dissects into the intestinal wall from the intestinal lumen or the lungs by the mediastinum because of increases in pressure, such as bowel obstruction and emphysema.
- Gas-forming bacteria enter the submucosa through mucosal tears or increased mucosal permeability and produce gas within the intestinal wall.

### Benign and Life-threatening Causes

- Benign causes
  - Pulmonary: COPD, asthma, pulmonary fibrosis, increased PEEP, cystic fibrosis
  - Systemic disease: Scleroderma, SLE, AIDS
  - Intestinal causes: Pyloric stenosis, enteritis, colitis, peptic ulcers, bowel obstruction
  - Iatrogenic: Barium enema, endoscopy, bowel surgery
  - Medications: Corticosteroids, lactulose, sorbitol, chemotherapy
  - Organ transplantation and graft-versus-host disease
- Life-threatening causes
  - Vascular: Mesenteric vascular disease, vasculitis
  - Intestinal: Obstruction/strangulation, enteritis, colitis, corrosive agent ingestion, toxic megacolon
  - Trauma
  - Organ transplantation most specifically bone marrow transplant
  - Collagen vascular disease

### CT Findings

- Linear or bubbly gas in the bowel wall
- Benign findings: pneumatosis only, without peritoneal signs on physical examination
- Life-threatening finding: pneumatosis with bowel wall thickening, dilated bowel, arterial or venous occlusion, ascites, and/or hepatic portal or portomesenteric venous gas

### Portal Venous Gas Versus Pneumobilia

- Portal venous gas: tubular branching lucencies extending to the periphery of the liver
- Pneumobilia: lucencies remain central

## Management

Treatment of underlying cause.

## Further Reading

Ho L, Paulson E, Thompson W. Pneumatosis intestinalis in the adult: benign to Life-threatening causes. *Am J Radiol.* 2007;188:1604–1613

## History

▸ 66-year-old male with nausea and vomiting.

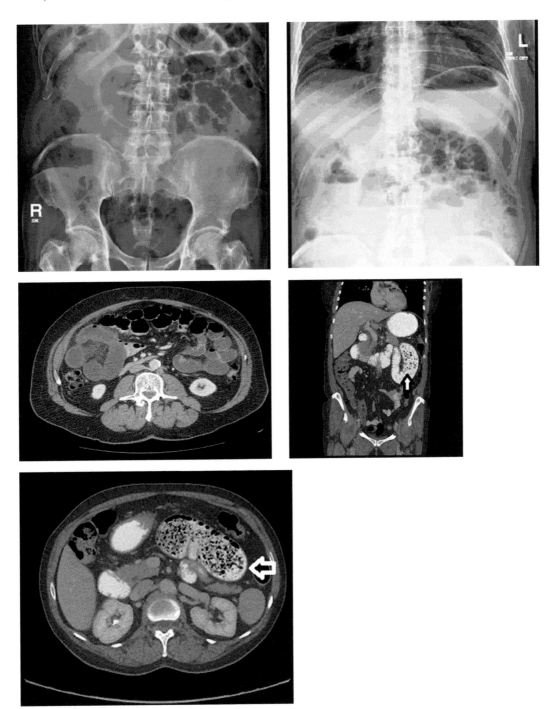

**Figures 130.1–130.5**

# Case 130  Small Bowel Obstruction

## Findings

▸ Supine AP view of the abdomen demonstrates multiple abnormally dilated loops of small bowel.
▸ Upright PA view of the abdomen demonstrates multiple air-fluid levels.
▸ Axial CT with intravenous and oral contrast demonstrates multiple loops of bowel with stranding in the mesentery in the right abdomen. The colon is normal in caliber.
▸ Coronal CT showing fecalization of a loop of small bowel.
▸ Axial CT showing fecalization of a loop of small bowel.

## Teaching Points

### Key Radiographic Findings

▸ Small bowel distention, with maximal dilated loops averaging 36 mm in diameter and exceeding 50% of the caliber of the largest visible colon loop.
▸ Presence of more than two air-fluid levels, air-fluid levels wider than 2.5 cm, and air-fluid levels differing more than 2 cm in height from one another within the same small bowel loop

### Key CT Findings

▸ Presence of dilated small bowel loops, with diameter >25 mm from outer wall to outer wall, proximal to normal caliber or collapse loops distally.
▸ Presence of small bowel feces sign (Figure 130.4)
▸ Sometimes obvious cause of small bowel obstruction, such as hernia or mass, is found; if none found, cause is likely adhesions with a history of surgery
▸ CT signs of bowel at risk
  ▪ Thickened and enhancing bowel wall (caused by venous and lymphatic obstruction)
  ▪ Portal venous gas (implies ischemic bowel)
  ▪ Free air (implies perforated bowel)
▸ Strangulated bowel: bowel obstructed at two points

## Causes of Small Bowel Obstruction

### Extrinsic Causes

▸ Adhesions, most common cause
▸ Internal and external hernias, second most common cause
▸ Endometriosis

### Intrinsic Causes

▸ Inflammatory, such as Crohn disease and eosinophilic gastroenteritis
▸ Neoplasm such as GIST, adenocarcinoma, and metastasis
▸ Hematoma from trauma and anticoagulation therapy
▸ Intussusception

### Intraluminal Causes

▸ Gallstones
▸ Bezoars
▸ Foreign bodies

## Management

▸ Bowel rest with gastric decompression with nasogastric tube.
▸ If obstruction does not resolve with conservative management, surgical intervention is warranted

## History

▶ Fever, nausea, and right lower quadrant pain.

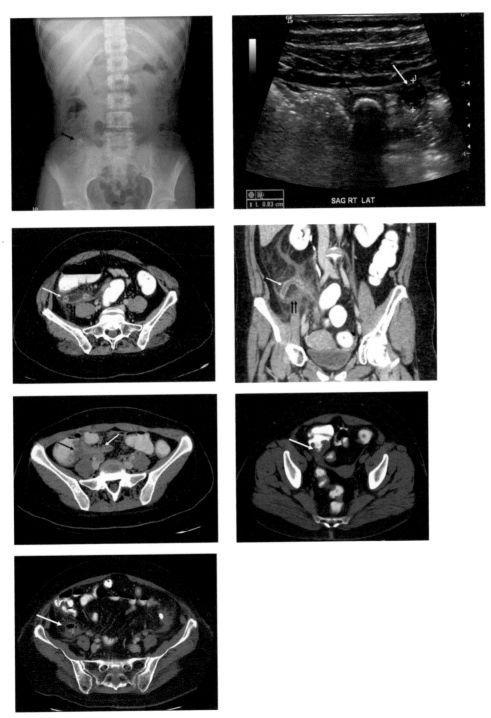

**Figures 131.1–131.7**

# Case 131   Appendicitis

## Findings

▶ Frontal abdominal radiograph (Figure 131.1) and right lower quadrant ultrasound (Figure 131.2) demonstrate an appendicolith (black arrow) in the right lower quadrant with an enlarged appendix (white arrow).

▶ Axial (Figure 131.3) and coronal reformat (Figure 131.4) images from a contrast-enhanced CT scan of the abdomen show a thickened appendix with hyperemic walls (white arrow). There is also periappendiceal fat-stranding and free fluid (double black arrows).

## Differential Diagnosis

▶ Mesenteric infarct
▶ Epiploic appendicitis
▶ Mesenteric adenitis
▶ Cecal diverticulitis
▶ Crohn disease
▶ Terminal ileitis
▶ Typhlitis
▶ Appendiceal mucocele

## Teaching Points

▶ Appendicitis is the most common surgical emergency in childhood
▶ Ultrasound has variable accuracy in its detection of appendicitis because of technical factors but is a reasonable first examination in children, pregnancy, and thin patients
▶ Ultrasonographic findings in appendicitis include appendiceal diameter >6–7 mm, appendicolith, free fluid, and bowel wall thickening
▶ CT is both highly sensitive and specific for the detection of appendicitis. CT findings of appendicitis include appendiceal diameter >6–7 mm, hyperemia, bowel wall thickening including the cecal bar sign (Figure 131.5) and cecal arrowhead sign (Figure 131.6), fat stranding, lack of intraluminal air and contrast, and free fluid
▶ MRI has been shown to be of value in the diagnosis of appendicitis in pregnancy without exposing the fetus to ionizing radiation
▶ Most complications of appendicitis are secondary to perforation (Figure 131.7) and include abscess formation, peritonitis, sepsis, bowel obstruction, infertility, and death

## Management

▶ Surgical evaluation for appendectomy or drainage and antibiotics, if perforated

## Further Readings

Leite NP, et al. CT evaluation of appendicitis and its complications: imaging techniques and key diagnostic findings. *AJR Am J Roentgenol.* 2005;185(2):406–417.

Sivit CJ, et al. When appendicitis is suspected in children. *RadioGraphics.* 2001;21(1):247–262.

Cobben LP, et al. MRI for clinically suspected appendicitis during pregnancy. *AJR Am J Roentgenol.* 2004;183(3):671–675.

**History**

► None

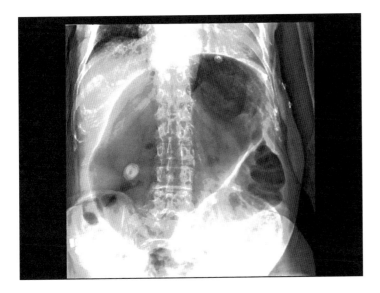

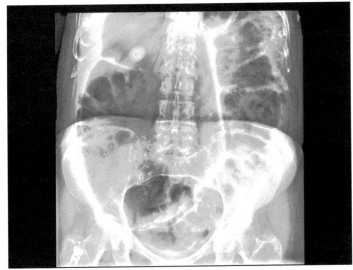

**Figures 132.1–132.2**

# Case 132  Cecal Volvulus

## Findings

### Radiograph

▶ Prominent focal loop of air-distended large bowel with its axis extending from the right lower quadrant to the left upper quadrant.
▶ Small bowel dilatation and air-fluid levels may be present depending on acuity.

### CT

▶ Severe colonic dilation with decompressed colon distally.
▶ Dilation and fecalization of small bowel.
▶ Transition point in the colon.
▶ "Whirl sign" toward the root of the mesentery where it twists on itself.
▶ "Beak-like" tapering of the colon at the level of the volvulus.
▶ "Split wall" sign shows apparent separation of cecal wall by adjacent mesenteric fat.

## Differential Diagnosis

▶ Sigmoid volvulus
▶ Ogilvie syndrome (pseudo-obstruction)
▶ Toxic megacolon
▶ Colonic obstruction

## Teaching Points

▶ Usually presents with colicky abdominal pain, abdominal distention, and vomiting.
▶ Different from "cecal bascule," which refers to an abnormal location of the cecum in the mid-abdomen resulting from the cecum folding up on itself without associated rotation along its axis. This can occur when the cecum is loosely attached to the mesentery and is excessively mobile.

## Management

▶ Reduction with enema may be attempted.
▶ Treatment is usually surgical.

### Further Readings

Peterson CM, Anderson JS, Hara AK, Carenza JW, Menias CO. Volvulus of the gastrointestinal tract: appearances at multimodality imaging. *RadioGraphics*. 2009;29(5):1281–1293.
Rosenblat JM, Rozenblit AM, Wolf EL, DuBrow RA, Den EI, Levsky JM. Findings of cecal volvulus at CT. *Radiology*. 2010;256(1):169–175. PubMed PMID: 20574094.

## History

▶ 61-year-old male with left lower quadrant pain.

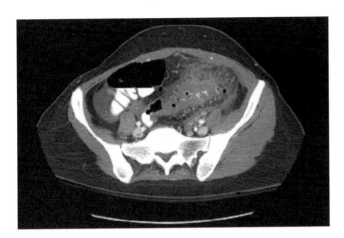

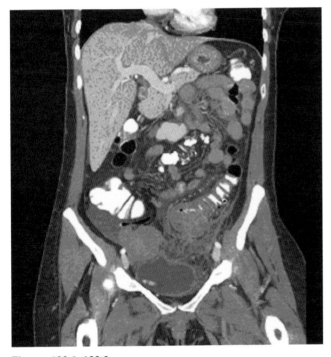

**Figures 133.1–133.2**

# Case 133  Diverticulitis

### Findings

- ▶ A segment of large bowel with wall thickening and associated fat stranding.
- ▶ Diverticula are seen in the vicinity.

### Differential Diagnosis

Segmental colitis from infectious, inflammatory, or ischemic etiology

### Teaching Points

- ▶ Common condition in Western society because of diet poor in fiber.
- ▶ Affects 5%–10% of people >45 years old and 80% of people >85 years of age.
- ▶ Manifests as outpouchings in the intestinal wall.
- ▶ Most common location is in the sigmoid.
- ▶ Caused by diverticulum occluded by stool, inflammation, or food debris leading to microperforation of the diverticulum and surrounding inflammation.
- ▶ CT findings of diverticulitis include segmental wall thickening, enhancement, adjacent fat stranding, and presence of diverticula.
- ▶ Complications include abscess, colovesicular and entero fistulas, perforation, and stricture formation.

### Management

- ▶ Intravenous or oral antibiotics
- ▶ Percutaneous drainage of abscess
- ▶ Surgical management of fistulas, perforation, and strictures.

### Further Reading

Horton K, Corl F, Fishman E. CT evaluation of the colon: inflammatory disease. *RadioGraphics.* 2000;20:399–418.

## History

▸ 32-year-old female presents with crampy abdominal pain.

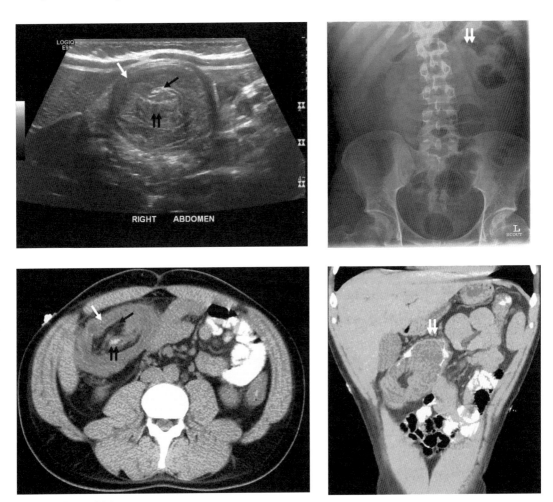

**Figures 134.1–134.4**

# Case 134  Intussusception

## Findings

▶ Transverse ultrasound image of the right abdomen (Figure 134.1) demonstrates a "target sign" with an isoechoic layer of outer bowel (the intussuscepiens, white arrow); a hyperechoic layer of mesenteric fat (black arrow); and a somewhat hypoechoic layer of inner bowel (the intussusceptum, double black arrows). These findings were confirmed with a contrast-enhanced CT (Figure 134.3).

▶ Frontal radiograph of the abdomen (Figure 134.2) shows a soft tissue mass (the intussusceptum, double white arrows) in the mid-abdomen. This finding was also confirmed with coronal reformatted images from a contrast-enhanced CT (Figure 134.4).

## Differential Diagnosis

▶ Idiopathic
▶ Primary bowel tumors (both benign and malignant)
▶ Enteritis
▶ Lymphoma
▶ Meckel diverticulum
▶ Metastatic disease

## Teaching Points

▶ Intussusception is the peristaltic telescoping of a loop of bowel with its mesenteric fat (the intussusceptum) into the lumen of a contiguous loop of bowel (the intussuscepiens). Most intussusceptions occur in children, commonly between the ages of 6 months and 2 years.

▶ Intussusception is most commonly idiopathic in children, whereas most intussusceptions in adults are secondary to "lead points," such as primary bowel tumors, lymphoma, or metastatic disease.

▶ Ultrasound is the initial imaging modality of choice for the diagnosis of intussusception, which can demonstrate a "target sign" (Figure 134.1) or a "pseudokidney sign" where there are multiple layers of hyperechogenicity and hypoechogenicity within a reniform mass.

▶ Radiographic signs of intussusception include a soft tissue mass (Figure 134.2), signs of obstruction, and a "crescent sign" where there is lucent air surrounding a soft tissue mass in the abdomen.

▶ CT can also demonstrate the "target sign" (Figure 134.3) and aid in the search of possible "lead points."

## Management

▶ Image-guided barium or air enema to reduce the intussusception with a surgeon on stand-by in case of bowel perforation.

### Further Readings

del-Pozo G, Albillos JC, Tejedor D, et al. Intussusception in children: current concepts in diagnosis and enema reduction. *RadioGraphics*. 1999;19(2):299–319.

Kim YH, Blake MA, Harisinghani MG, et al. Adult intestinal intussusception: CT appearances and identification of a causative lead point. *RadioGraphics*. 2006;26(3):733–744.

## History

▶ Abdominal pain and distention.

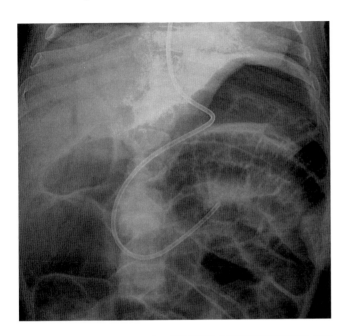

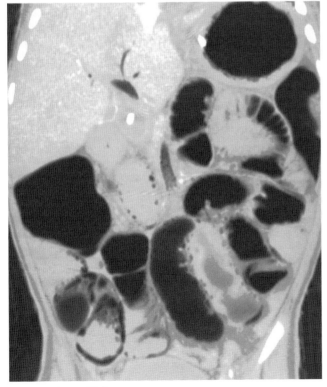

**Figures 135.1–135.2**

# Case 135 Small Bowel Ischemia

## Findings

### Radiographs

- ► Bowel dilation with air-fluid levels
- ► Pneumatosis intestinalis
- ► Portal venous gas

### Contrast-enhanced Computed Tomography

- ► SMA, SMV, or other mesenteric vessel occlusion (most specific sign)
- ► Mesenteric or portal venous gas
- ► Decreased bowel wall enhancement caused by decreased arterial flow
- ► Bowel wall thickening (>3mm) caused by edema, hemorrhage, or superimposed infection
- ► Bowel dilation with air-fluid levels
- ► Mesenteric fat infiltration caused by edema (more common with venous occlusion)
- ► Pneumatosis

## Differential Diagnosis

- ► Infectious enteritis
- ► Shock bowel
- ► Inflammatory bowel disease (e.g., Crohn disease)
- ► Fibrosis mesenteritis

## Teaching Points

- ► Presentation
  - ▪ Acute ischemia: sudden onset of abdominal pain, vomiting, diarrhea
  - ▪ Chronic ischemia: chronic, intermittent abdominal pain (intestinal angina)
- ► Etiology
  - ▪ Vascular occlusion (atherosclerosis, thromboembolic)
  - ▪ Bowel herniation or closed loop obstruction
  - ▪ Hypercoagulable states
  - ▪ Inflammatory (e.g., vasculitis)
  - ▪ Hypoperfusion (e.g., sepsis, hypovolemia)
  - ▪ Drugs (e.g., cocaine)
- ► Occlusion of the SMA or SMV is the most specific sign
  - ▪ Arterial occlusion may be complete or partial

## Management

- ► Surgical
  - ▪ Exploratory laparotomy with resection of nonviable bowel +/- vascular bypass
- ► Endovascular recanalization of vascular occlusion
- ► Anticoagulation for venous thrombosis

## Further Readings

Furukawa A, Kanasaki S, Kono N, et al. CT diagnosis of acute mesenteric ischemia from various causes. *AJR Am J Roentgenol.* 2009 Feb;192(2):408–416.

Wiesner W, Khurana B, Ji H, et al. CT of acute bowel ischemia. *Radiology.* 2003;226:635.

## History

▶ None.

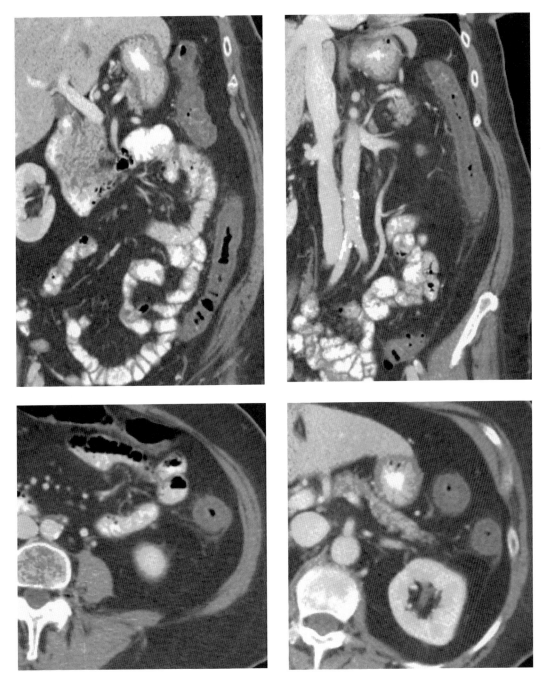

**Figures 136.1–136.4**

# Case 136  Ischemic Colitis

## Findings

### Radiograph

▶ "Thumbprinting" secondary to bowel wall edema
▶ Dilated loops of bowel secondary to ileus
▶ Pneumatosis or signs of portal venous air in the liver
▶ Free air if perforated

### CT

▶ Wall thickening within a vascular territory
▶ Low-density bowel wall resulting in a "target sign"
▶ Pneumatosis or portal venous air
▶ Signs of vascular occlusion involving the SMA or SMV.

## Differential Diagnosis

▶ Infectious colitis (pseudomembranous colitis "pancolitis")
▶ Inflammatory colitis
▶ Neoplastic (lymphoma can have associated lymphadenopathy)
▶ Radiation colitis (geographic involvement in the area of the radiation port)
▶ In immunocompromised individuals consider graft-versus-host disease or infections, such as cytomegalovirus

## Teaching Points

▶ Symptoms include abdominal pain, bloody diarrhea. In severe cases with perforation, it may present as an acute abdomen.
▶ Causes include arterial occlusion (atherosclerosis or embolic disease); venous thrombosis (hypercoagulable state); and hypotension/shock.
▶ Demonstrates a vascular distribution when caused by arterial occlusion.
  ▪ Superior mesenteric artery: from the cecum to the splenic flexure.
  ▪ Inferior mesenteric artery: splenic flexure to rectum.
▶ When caused by low-flow states findings may localize to watershed areas, such as the splenic flexure (Griffith point) or rectosigmoid junction (point of Sudeck).

## Management

▶ Anticoagulation and thrombolysis
▶ Surgical resection may be required in sever cases with perforation or peritonitis

## Further Readings

Balthazar EJ, Yen BC, Gordon RB. Ischemic colitis: CT evaluation of 54 cases. *Radiology*. 1999;211(2):381–388. PubMed PMID: 10228517.
Dahnert W. *Radiology Review Manual*, 6th edn. Lippincott, Williams & Wilkins, Philadelphia, PA, 2007.

## History

▶ 21-year-old male with bloody diarrhea after course of amoxicillin for ear infection.

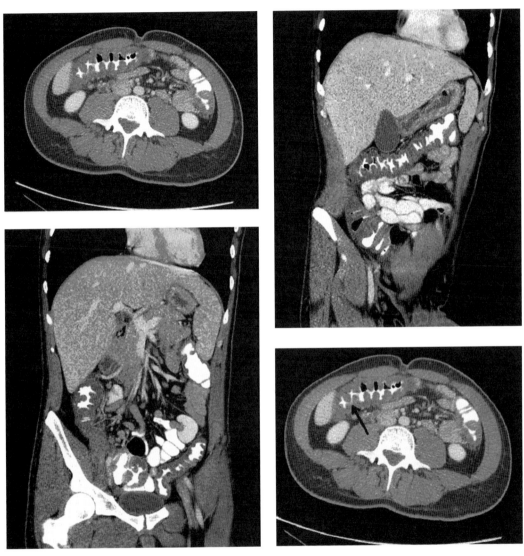

**Figures 137.1–137.4**

# Case 137  Pseudomembranous Colitis

### Findings

▶ Axial and coronal CT with intravenous and oral contrast demonstrating thickening of the entire colonic wall consistent with pancolitis.

### Differential Diagnosis

▶ Pancolitis from inflammatory, infectious, or ischemic cause.

### Teaching Points

▶ Causal agent: *Clostridium difficile*, producing toxins A and B.
▶ Proliferation of *C. difficile* caused by insult to the normal flora in the intestinal tract from antibiotics or chemotherapy.
▶ Pseudomembranes are the result of fibrin, inflammatory cells, and cellular debris adhering to intestinal walls.
▶ Results in watery diarrhea, abdominal pain, fever, leukocytosis, sepsis, toxic megacolon colonic perforation, and even death.
▶ CT findings: Diffuse colonic thickening (pancolitis); pericolonic stranding and edema; ascites; and the "accordion" sign (Figure 137.4), which is the appearance of oral contrast material between thickened intestinal folds.

### Management

▶ Cessation of antibiotics, oral or intravenous metronidazole, oral vancomycin, attempts to replenish normal intestinal flora.

Further Reading

Kilpatrick I, Greenberg H. Gastrointestinal imaging: evaluating the CT diagnosis of *Clostridium difficile* colitis: should CT guide therapy? *Am J Radiol.* 2001;176:635–639.

## History

▶ 68-year-old male with IBD presenting with fever, abdominal pain, and bloody diarrhea.

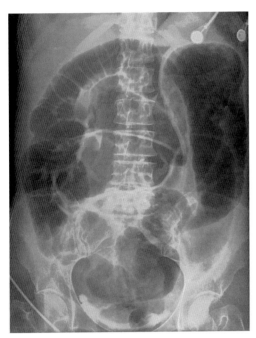 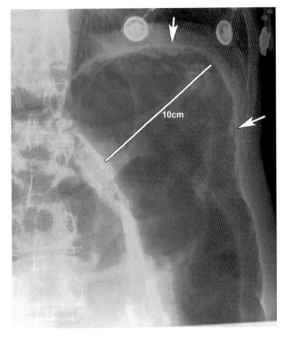

**Figures 138.1–138.2**

# Case 138  Toxic Megacolon

## Findings

### Radiograph

▸ Marked colonic dilation (mean diameter 8–9 cm)
▸ Serial radiographs with progressive dilation
▸ Transverse colon most common
▸ Loss of normal haustral folds
▸ "Pseudopolyps" and thumbprinting caused by mucosal edema
▸ Pneumatosis ± pneumoperitoneum

### CT

▸ Colonic dilation filled with air and fluid
▸ Loss of normal mucosal pattern with irregular nodular contour
▸ Pneumatosis ± pneumoperitoneum
▸ Ascites ± mesenteric abscess

## Differential Diagnosis

▸ Distal colon obstruction
▸ Adynamic ileus (Ogilvie syndrome)
▸ Sigmoid volvulus

## Teaching Points

▸ Severe life-threatening complication of inflammatory bowel disease or infectious colitis
▸ Ulcerative colitis most common
▸ Transverse colon most commonly affected
▸ Progressive dilation on serial radiographs should raise suspicion
▸ Dilated colon (8–9 cm) compared with normal diameter of 5–6 cm

## Management

▸ Colectomy

## Further Readings

Imbriaco M, Balthazar EJ. Toxic megacolon: role of CT in evaluation and detection of complications. *Clin Imaging.* 2001;25:349.
Thoeni RF, Cello JP. CT imaging of colitis. *Radiology.* 2006;240:623.

## History

▶ 40-year-old male with acute myelocytic leukemia presenting with abdominal pain status postchemotherapy.

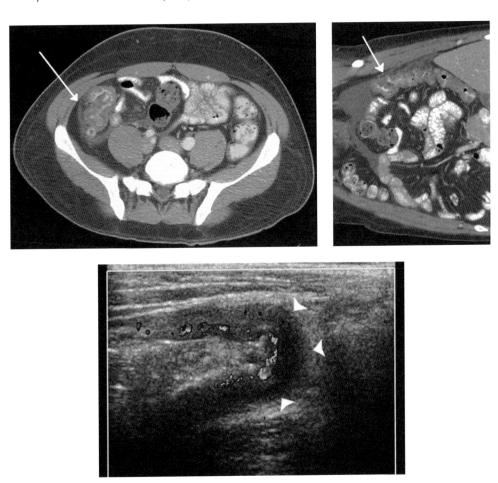

**Figures 139.1–139.3**

# Case 139  Typhlitis

## Findings

### Radiography

▶ Nonspecific and may be normal

▶ Possible findings include cecal thumbprinting, distention of cecum and/or small bowel loops, soft tissue mass in the right lower quadrant with paucity of right colonic gas, pneumatosis or free air

### CT

▶ Circumferential low-density cecal wall thickening and/or distention with adjacent fat stranding (arrows)

▶ High-density hemorrhage may be present in cecal wall

▶ Inflammation may extend to the appendix, ascending colon, and/or ileum

▶ Possible complications include hemorrhage, pneumoperitoneum, abscess, pneumatosis, portal venous gas, and necrosis

### US

▶ Thickened bowel wall with hyperechogenic mucosa, decreased peristalsis, and hyperemia on color imaging (arrowheads)

## Differential Diagnosis

▶ Appendicitis

▶ Infectious colitis, including pseudomembranous colitis

▶ Ischemic colitis

▶ Inflammatory bowel disease

▶ Toxic megacolon

▶ Ogilvie syndrome

▶ Mesenteric adenitis

## Teaching Points

▶ Etiology

  ▪ Moderate neutropenia is invariably present, leading to compromised host defense

  ▪ Other etiologic factors include mucosal injury from cytotoxic drugs; cecal distention causing impaired perfusion; antibiotics and steroids, which alter normal gut flora; and bacterial or fungal invasion of the bowel wall

▶ Epidemiology

  ▪ Neutropenia leading to typhlitis is most commonly a result of cytotoxic chemotherapeutic agents

  ▪ Other causes of neutropenia include myelodysplastic syndromes, multiple myeloma, aplastic anemia, lymphoma, AIDS, and immunosuppression after solid organ or bone marrow transplantation

▶ Presentation

  ▪ Onset of symptoms is typically within 10–14 days of chemotherapy

  ▪ Symptoms include right lower quadrant abdominal pain, fever, watery or bloody diarrhea, nausea, vomiting, and abdominal distention

## Management

▶ Conservative management includes bowel rest and IV broad-spectrum antibiotics

▶ Surgery is indicated with free perforation, abscess formation, refractory hemorrhage, or failure to respond to medical management; options include cecostomy, hemicolectomy or total colectomy, and/or loop ileostomy

## History

▸ 18-year-old with scrotal pain.

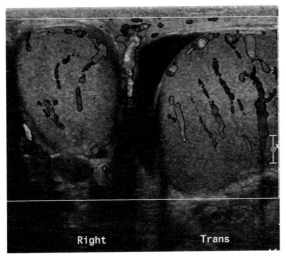

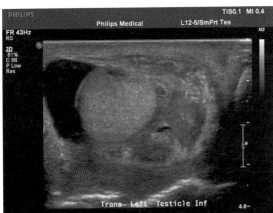

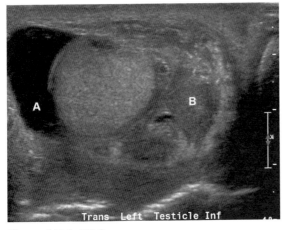

**Figures 140.1–140.3**

# Case 140  Epididymitis/Orchitis

## Findings

▶ Ultrasound of the scrotum demonstrates increased color flow in the left testicle when compared with the right. Note the reactive hydrocele (Figure 140.1).

▶ Ultrasound of the left hemiscrotum demonstrates a reactive hydrocele (Figure 140.2) and a heterogeneous echogenic focus (Figure 140.3) at the base of the testicle, which represents an enlarged, inflamed epididymis.

## Differential Diagnosis

▶ Epididymo-orchitis

▶ Epididymitis

▶ Orchitis

▶ Testicular trauma

## Teaching Points

▶ Epididymitis is the most common cause of nontraumatic acute scrotal pain in adult men.

▶ Acute epididymitis is a clinical syndrome of pain, swelling, and inflammation of the epididymis. Fever, dysuria, or urethral discharge may accompany signs of epididymitis.

▶ It is usually caused by bacterial spread from the urethra, prostate, or bladder. It is commonly linked to *Chlamydia trachomatis* or *Neisseria gonorrhea* in sexually active men; however, urinary tract or *Escherichia coli* infections can cause epididymitis in other settings.

▶ Symptoms of orchitis can mimic testicular torsion and include pain, swelling, and hematuria. Orchitis associated with sexually transmitted bacterial infection can involve the epididymis.

▶ Orchitis can be seen among adolescent boys during active mumps.

## Management

▶ Antibiotic therapy in bacterial cases. Antibiotics are not suggested in viral causes.

▶ Anti-inflammatory drugs.

### Further Readings

Aso C, Enríquez G, Fité M, et al. Gray-scale and color Doppler sonography of scrotal disorders in children: an update. *Radiographics*. 2005 Sep-Oct;25(5):1197–1214.

Blaivas M, Sierzenski P, Lambert M. Emergency evaluation of patients presenting with acute scrotum using bedside ultrasonography. *Acad Emerg Med*. 2001;8(1):90–93.

Trojian TH, Lishnak TS, Heiman D. Epididymitis and orchitis: an overview. *Am Fam Physician*. 2009;79(7):583–587.

## History

▶ 42-year-old female with fever, altered mental status, and abdominal pain.

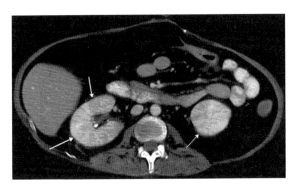 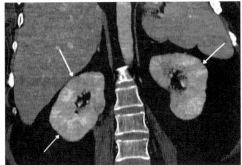

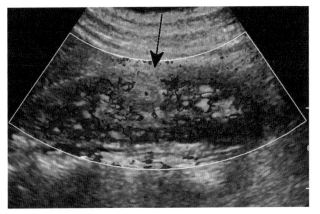

**Figures 141.1–141.3**

# Case 141   Pyelonephritis

## Findings

### CT

► Striated nephrogram: wedge-shaped areas of alternating hyperenhancement and hypoenhancement (Figures 141.1 and 141.2, white arrows); best seen during excretory phase
► Enlarged, edematous kidney with loss of corticomedullary differentiation
► Perinephric fat stranding and thickening of Gerota facia
► Hydronephrosis if obstructed
► Emphysematous pyelonephritis: bubbles or streaky foci of intraparenchymal gas
► Pyelitis: urothelial thickening/enhancement of the collecting system with normal renal parenchyma
► Emphysematous pyelitis: pyelitis with foci of gas within the collecting system

### US

► Frequently normal
► Peripheral wedge-shaped hyperechoic or hypoechoic foci
► Loss of corticomedullary differentiation
► Focal area of hypoperfusion on power Doppler (Figure 141.3, black arrow)
► Focal bacterial nephritis may appear mass-like
► Gas may be seen as echogenic foci with posterior "dirty shadowing"

### Nuclear Medicine

► Tc-99m DMSA scintigraphy shows focal or diffuse photopenia
► Highly sensitive and preferred in pediatric patients; nonspecific in adults
► Cannot distinguish between pyelonephritis, abscess, cyst, infarct, or tumor

## Differential Diagnosis

► Renal infarct
► Ureteral obstruction
► Trauma
► Renal vein thrombosis
► Hypotension
► Intratubular obstruction
► Lymphoma

## Teaching Points

► Etiology
  ▪ Bacterial invasion of the renal parenchyma and pelvis with tubular obstruction, interstitial edema, and vasospasm
  ▪ Usually gram-negative organisms from ascending infection
► Complications
  ▪ Complications are more common with diabetes, chronic renal disease, sickle cell disease, renal transplant, and AIDS and other immunocompromised states
  ▪ Emphysematous pyelonephritis is a surgical emergency that usually occurs in patients with poorly controlled diabetes and represents necrotizing infection involving renal parenchyma
  ▪ Other complications include abscess formation, acute renal failure, sepsis, and scarring

## Management

► Antibiotics for noncomplicated pyelonephritis
► Nephrectomy for emphysematous pyelonephritis
► Emergent percutaneous drainage if obstructed

Case 142

History

None

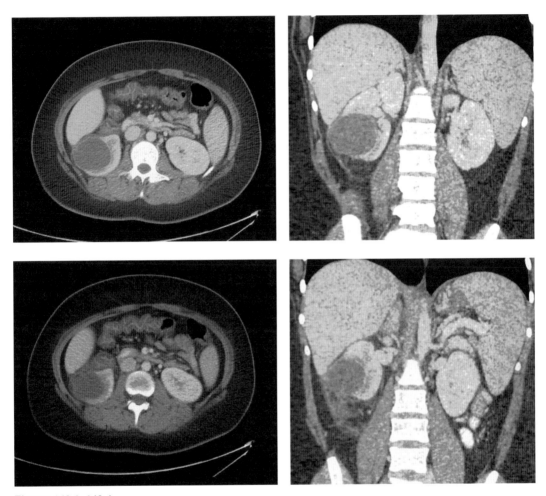

Figures 142.1–142.4

307

# Case 142  Renal Abscess

## Findings

### CT

- ▶ Low-attenuation mass with a thick, enhancing, irregular wall
- ▶ Surrounding fat stranding
- ▶ May contain foci of air internally
- ▶ Lack of central enhancement
- ▶ Possible hypoenhancement of the surrounding renal parenchyma
- ▶ May demonstrate perinephric extension

### US

- ▶ Well-defined heterogeneous area of hypoenhancement
- ▶ No internal flow
- ▶ May demonstrate "dirty shadowing" if there are internal foci of air

### MRI

- ▶ T1 hypointense
- ▶ T2 hyperintense
- ▶ May demonstrate wall enhancement

## Differential Diagnosis

- ▶ Renal cell carcinoma
- ▶ Metastasis
- ▶ Lymphoma
- ▶ Hemorrhagic or infected renal cyst

## Teaching Points

- ▶ Presents with fever, chills, dysuria, and flank pain
- ▶ May rupture into the collecting system or into the perinephric space

## Management

- ▶ Antibiotic therapy and drainage
- ▶ Medical antibiotic therapy alone may be appropriate if the abscess is small

Further Readings

Craig WD, Wagner BJ, Travis MD. Pyelonephritis: radiologic-pathologic review. *RadioGraphics*. 2008;28(1):255–277; quiz 327–328. PubMed PMID: 18203942.

Kawashima A, Sandler CM, Goldman SM, Raval BK, Fishman EK. CT of renal inflammatory disease. *RadioGraphics*. 1997;17(4):851–866; discussion 867–8. PubMed PMID: 9225387.

## History

▶ Left flank pain.

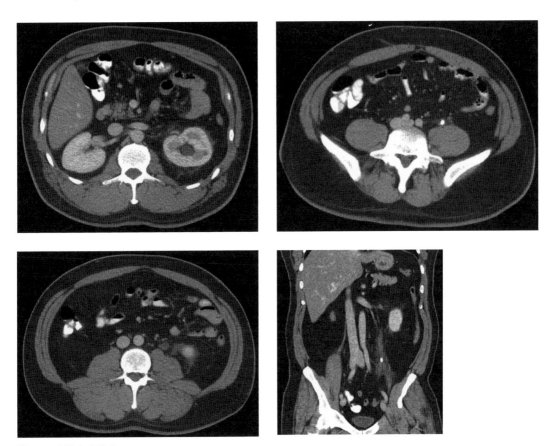

**Figures 143.1–143.4**

# Case 143  Ureteral Stone

## Findings

▶ Asymetric hydroureteronephrosis with perinephric stranding and fluid and radiopaque obstructing ureteral calculus. Asymetric delayed renal enhancement may be seen on contrast-enhanced scans.

▶ Approximately 77% of ureteral stones are surrounded by a rim of soft tissue knows as the "soft tissue rim sign," which assists in differention from phleboliths.

▶ Rescanning in the prone position may help differentiate between passed stones that fall anteriorly and stones within the ureterovesicular junction that do not.

▶ Approximately 50% of stones are not visible on abdominal radiographs.

## Teaching Points

▶ Calcium stones acount for 75% of renal calculi
▶ Other main types of stones are
  ▪ Struvite (magnesium ammonium phosphate)
    ▪ 15% of renal calculi
    ▪ Associated with chronic urinary tract infection
    ▪ Usual organisms include *Proteus*, *Pseudomonas*, and *Klebsiella* species
    ▪ Stones involving the renal pelvis and extending into two or more calyces are knows as staghorn calculi.
  ▪ Uric acid
    ▪ 6% of renal calculi
    ▪ Associated with high purine intake, or malignancy
    ▪ 25% of patients have gout
  ▪ Cystine
    ▪ 2% of renal calculi
    ▪ Caused by intrinsic metabolic defect resulting in failure of renal tubular absorbtion of cystine
▶ Size of stone important predictor of spontaneous passage
  ▪ Less that 4 mm in diameter has 80% chance of sponatneous passage
  ▪ 5–7 mm in diameter has 60% chance of spontaneous passage
  ▪ Larger that 8 mm in diameter has 20% chance of spontaneous passage
▶ Forniceal rupture
  ▪ Caused by increased renal pelvic pressure
  ▪ Characterized by significant amount of perinephric fluid or spillage of opacified urine into perinephric space
  ▪ Spares kidney from further damage by releasing built-up intrapelvic pressure
  ▪ Patient may report sudden resolution of pain

## Management

▶ Small stones with mild hydronephrosis may be treated with pain control and observation.
▶ Larger stones or patients with intractable pain may require drainage with ureteral stent or percutaneous nephrostomy.
▶ Evidence of infected hydronephrosis requires hospital admission and prompt drainage.

## Further Reading

Dalrymple NC, Casford B, Raiken DP, et al. Pearls and pitfalls in the diagnosis of ureterolisthiasis with unenhanced helical CT. *Radiographics*. 2000;20(2):439–447.

## History

▸ 40 year old with generalized pelvic pain.

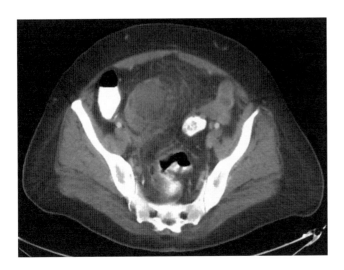

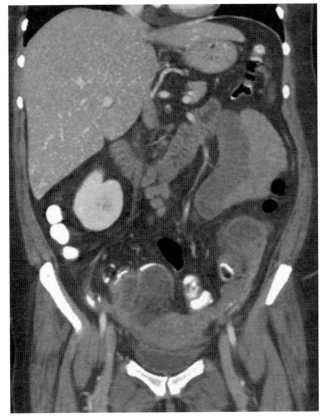

**Figures 144.1–144.2**

# Case 144   Tubo-Ovarian Abscess/Pelvic Inflammatory Disease

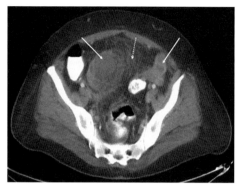 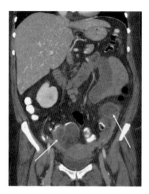

**Figures 144.3–144.4**

## Findings

### CT

- ▸ Distended thick-walled fallopian tube(s)
- ▸ Enlarged edematous ovaries
- ▸ Tubo-ovarian/pelvic abscess (solid arrows)
- ▸ Inflammatory stranding surrounding pelvic structures (dashed arrow)
- ▸ Free pelvic fluid (simple or complex)

### US

- ▸ Increased echogenicity of pelvic fat
- ▸ Distended serpiginous fallopian tube(s) with fluid and/or debris
- ▸ Enlarged adjacent ovary
- ▸ Multilocular, complex, thick-walled, cystic adnexal mass
- ▸ Surrounding hyperemia with low resistive flow

## Differential Diagnosis

- ▸ Hemorrhagic ovarian cyst (± rupture)
- ▸ Endometriosis
- ▸ Ovarian neoplasm
- ▸ Pelvic abscess of different etiology (e.g., diverticulitis, appendicitis, Crohn disease)

## Teaching Points

- ▸ Presentation
  - ▪ Fever, abdominal/pelvic pain, vaginal discharge, cervical/adnexal tenderness
- ▸ Risk factors
  - ▪ Multiple sexual partners, lower socioeconomic class, intrauterine contraceptive device, history of STD
- ▸ Pathology
  - ▪ Most commonly *Neisseria gonorrhea* or *Chlamydia trachomatis*, but 40% are polymicrobial
  - ▪ Results from untreated ascending vaginal infection that progresses to endometritis, salpingitis, and tubo-ovarian abscess

## Management

- ▸ Intrauterine contraceptive device removed if present, antibiotic therapy ± abscess drainage
- ▸ Can lead to infertility and ectopic pregnancies if not diagnosed and treated early

## Further Readings

Potter A, Chandrasekhar CA. et al. US and CT evaluation of acute pelvic pain of gynecologic origin in nonpregnant premenopausal patients. *RadioGraphics*. 2008;28:1645–1659.

Sam JW, Jacobs JE, Birnbaum BA. et al. Spectrum of CT findings in acute pyogenic pelvic inflammatory disease. *RadioGraphics*. 2002;22:1327–1334.

## History

▶ None

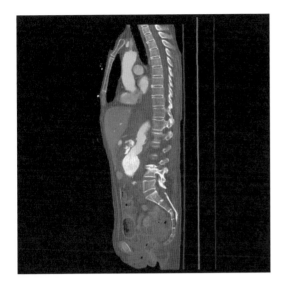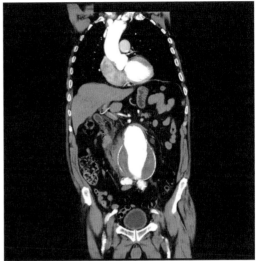

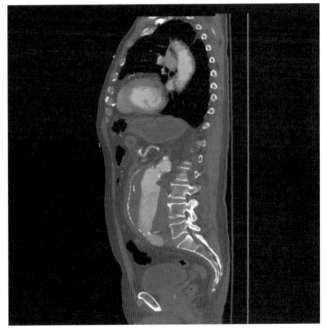

**Figures 145.1–145.3**

# Case 145  Abdominal Aortic Aneurysm (AAA Rupture)

## Findings

▶ Abdominal aortic aneurysm rupture with active extravasation
▶ Contained abdominal aortic aneurysm rupture: Coronal
▶ Contained abdominal aortic aneurysm: Sagittal

## Teaching Points

▶ Characterization of an aortic aneurysm
  ▪ Location
    ▪ Ascending
    ▪ Arch
    ▪ Descending
  ▪ Shape
    ▪ Fusiform
    ▪ Saccular
  ▪ Etiology
    ▪ Atherosclerotic
    ▪ Mycotic
    ▪ Traumatic
    ▪ Inflammatory
    ▪ Iatrogenic
    ▪ Congenital
▶ The wall stress is uniformly distributed in the nonaneurysmal aorta, whereas within an aortic aneurysm, regions of high and low stress distribution are present.
▶ CT allows precise measurement of aneurysm size and evaluation of disease extent.
▶ On average, an abdominal aortic aneurysm expands at a rate of 2–4 mm per year for aneurysms <4 cm, 2–5 mm for aneurysms 4–5 cm, and 3–7 mm for those >5 cm.
▶ The risk of rupture is size dependent with the risk being 2%, 10%, and 22% at 4 years, respectively.
▶ Most abdominal aortic aneurysms rupture into the retroperitoneum.
▶ Thoracic aortic aneurysm rupture may result in pericardial and/or pleural effusions and mediastinal hematoma.
▶ Aortic aneurysms may be complicated by dissection and distal embolization, which can cause bowel or extremity ischemia or infarction.
▶ CT is the modality of choice when evaluating patients for aneurysm leak. Signs of impending rupture
  ▪ Increased aneurysm size
  ▪ Low thrombus-to-lumen ration
  ▪ Hemorrhage into a mural thrombus
  ▪ Peripheral crescent-shaped area of high attenuation within the aneurysm
  ▪ Draping of the aneurysmal aorta over the vertebrae
  ▪ Noncontrast CT shows high attenuation surrounding the aorta with loss of the fat interface between the aortic wall and hematoma.
▶ Focal discontinuity in circumferential wall calcifications is more frequently observed in unstable or ruptured aneurysms.
▶ A true aneurysm involves all three wall layers: intima, media, and adventitia.
▶ A false aneurysm or pseudoaneurysm involves one or two wall layers.

## Management

▶ Endovascular aneurysm repair versus conventional open surgical repair
▶ Initial length of hospital stay is shorter for the patients undergoing endovascular aneurysm: however, these patients often have more frequent readmission for the treatment of procedure-related complications, chiefly endoleak.

## History

▶ None

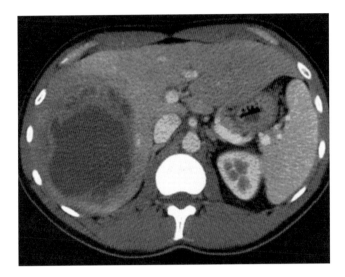

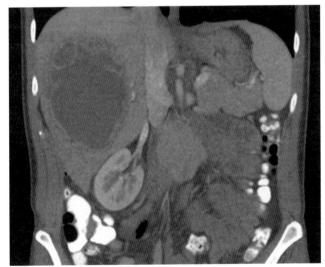

**Figures 146.1–146.2**

# Case 146  Liver Abscess

## Findings
### CT
► Peripherally enhancing lesions with central low density
► Lacy appearance with satellite lesions
► Often found in the dependent portion of right lobe
► May contain foci of gas

### US
► Poorly defined
► Variable internal echogenicity but often heterogeneous
► No central flow

### MRI
► Usually heterogeneous and T1 hypointense centrally
► Usually T2 hyperintense centrally
► Often demonstrates capsular enhancement

## Differential Diagnosis
► Metastatic disease
► Hepatocellular carcinoma
► Biliary cystadenoma/carcinoma
► Echinococcal cyst

## Teaching Points
► Presents with fever, chills, and upper abdominal pain.
► Rare in healthy individuals and usually seen in the setting of an immunocompromised patient.
► Look for diverticulitis, appendicitis, or other source of infection as a potential cause.
► In developing countries, parasitic abscesses are more common.

## Management
► Surgical consult and IR drainage.
► Medical antibiotic therapy alone may be appropriate if the abscess is small.

## Further Readings
Mortelé KJ, Segatto E, Ros PR. The infected liver: radiologic-pathologic correlation. *RadioGraphics*. 2004;24(4):937–955. PubMed PMID: 15256619.
Mortelé KJ, Ros PR. Cystic focal liver lesions in the adult: differential CT and MR imaging features. *RadioGraphics*. 2001;21(4):895–910. PubMed PMID: 11452064.

## History

▸ Right-sided pelvic pain.

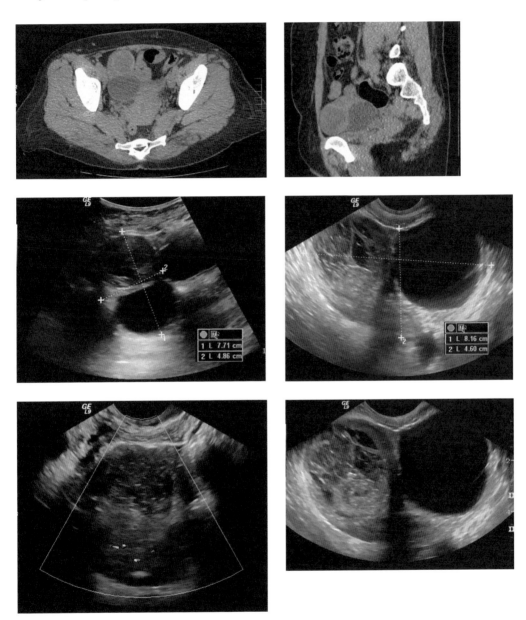

**Figures 147.1–147.6**

# Case 147 Adnexal Torsion

## Findings
- Enlarged (>5 cm), bulky-appearing ovary
- Frequently has an associated adnexal cyst or mass leading to increased size
- May see peritoneal fluid
- Ultrasound
  - Doppler flow may be absent or systolic-only
  - May see hypoechoic (edematous) central ovary with hemorrhagic areas; follicles may be displaced to the periphery
  - "Whirlpool" sign of a twisted vessel may be seen
- CT
  - Fallopian tube thickening
  - May see adnexal mass with twisted pedicle
  - May see deviation of the uterus to the torsed adnexa
- MR
  - Fallopian tube thickening
  - Heterogeneous ovarian parenchyma with hemorrhagic areas
  - May be able to narrow diagnosis of underlying ovarian lesion
  - Better delineation of blood products in lesion or peritoneum

## Differential Diagnosis
- Hemorrhagic ovarian cyst
- Adnexal mass (benign)
- Ovarian hyperstimulation syndrome in the context of infertility treatment
- Ectopic pregnancy

## Teaching Points
- Commonly occurs in reproductive-age females, and even more commonly during pregnancy.
- Most common underlying ovarian lesion is the mature cystic teratoma (dermoid cyst).
- Ovarian torsion is primarily a clinical diagnosis. Imaging features can suggest the diagnosis, but cannot rule it out and are rarely specific enough for definitive diagnosis.
- Presence of Doppler flow within the ovary is *not* sufficient to exclude torsion. Contrariwise, absence of measurable flow is suggestive, but not diagnostic.

## Management
- Classically, managed with salpingo-oophrectomy, usually laparoscopic out of concern for development of thromboembolism.
- More conservative ovary-sparing treatment with simple laparoscopic detorsion may be used in younger women.

Further Readings

Rha SE, Byun JY, Jung SE, et al. CT and MR imaging features of adnexal torsion. *RadioGraphics*. 2002;22(2):283–294.
Chang HC, Bhatt S, Dogra VS. Pearls and pitfalls in diagnosis of ovarian torsion. *RadioGraphics*. 2008;28(5):1355–1368; doi:10.1148/rg.285075130.

## History

▸ Pelvic pain, history of infertility.

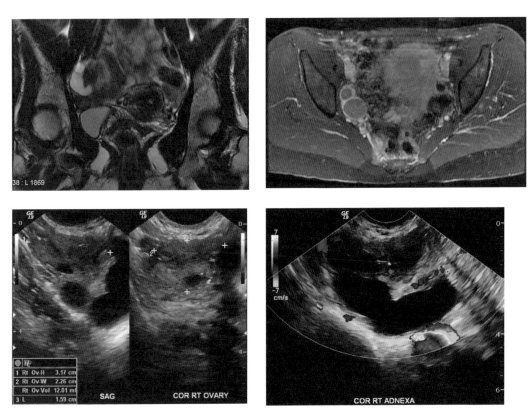

**Figures 148.1–148.4**

# Case 148  Hydrosalpinx

## Findings

### Ultrasound

- Hypoechoic tubular structure in the adnexa adjacent to the ovary
- Debris within the structure
- May see thickened longitudinal folds
- No flow seen within the structure

### MRI

- Dilated tubular structure, definitely separate from the ovary
- Clearer delineation of the tubular nature of the structure and its relationship to the ovary and uterus
- May see fluid-fluid level, suggestive of blood products
- Thickness of the tubal wall can be important distinguishing factor between inflammatory and noninflammatory etiologies

## Differential Diagnosis

- Hematosalpix versus hematosalpinx versus pyosalpinx
- Tubal ectopic pregnancy
- Tubo-ovarian abscess
- Peritoneal cyst
- Adnexal cystic lesion

## Teaching Points

- Etiology of hydrosalpinx is typically related to obstruction caused by adhesions or endometriosis.
- Echogenic debris within the tubular structure suggests the possibility of pyosalpinx. Thickened, enhancing tube wall is also suggestive of an inflammatory process.
- Thickened longitudinal folds are highly suggestive of hydrosalpinx associated with chronic inflammation.
- Carefully evaluate for a solid mass within the fluid-filled structure, which could represent an ectopic pregnancy or a fallopian tube adenocarcinoma.
- Can be associated with tubal factors for infertility, such as endometriosis or pelvic inflammatory disease.

## Management

- Management depends on underlying etiology: treatment of pelvic inflammatory disease, of endometriosis, of ectopic pregnancy, and so forth.
- In infertile patients, in vitro fertilization techniques may be used.

## Further Readings

Kim MK, Rha SE, Oh SN, et al. MR imaging findings of hydrosalpinx: a comprehensive review. *RadioGraphics.* 2009;29(2):495–507. doi:10.1148/rg.292085070.

Moyle PL, Kataoka MY, Nakai A, Takahata A, Reinhold C, Sala E. Nonovarian cystic lesions of the pelvis. *RadioGraphics.* 2010;30(4):921–938. doi:10.1148/rg.304095706.

Rezvani M, Shaaban AM. Fallopian tube disease in the nonpregnant patient. *RadioGraphics.* 2011;31(2):527–548. doi:10.1148/rg.312105090.

## History

▸ Abdominal pain.

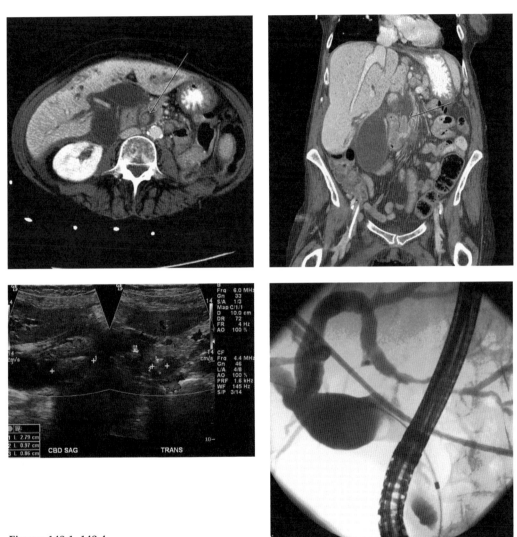

**Figures 149.1–149.4**

# Case 149 Choledocholithiasis (CBD Stone)

## Findings

▶ CT: Axial and coronal images, demonstrating dilated common bile duct (CBD) and dilated intrahepatic bile ducts. A round hyperdense lesion in the lumen of the distal CBD (arrow).

▶ US: A round echogenic structure with posterior acoustic shadowing in a dilated CBD.

▶ ERCP: demonstrating a dilated CBD, with a large filling defect.

## Differential Diagnosis

▶ CT findings: CBD stricture from benign or malignant cause (ampullary carcinoma, pancreatic adenocarcinoma), obstructed CBD from gallbladder sludge.

## Teaching Points

▶ Gallstones can migrate from the gallbladder lumen into the bile duct and be associated with biliary colic, jaundice, CBD obstruction, and hyperbilirubinemia and elevated alkaline phosphatase.

▶ The entire length of the CBD may not be visualized by ultrasound, making MRI/MRCP or ERCP useful adjunct modalities in further evaluation for choledocholithiasis.

▶ CBD stones may be occult on CT, depending on their size and composition.

▶ CBD stones are present in 10%–15% of patients with gallstones.

## Management

▶ If US demonstrates a stone, the patient should be referred for ERCP and definitive management with papillotomy, stone removal, and potential subsequent cholecystectomy.

▶ If US fails to demonstrate a stone, the patient may be referred for MRI/MRCP, or thin-slice CT with and without contrast as an alternative if an MRI cannot be obtained.

### Further Readings

Hanbidge AE, Buckler PM, O'Malley ME, et al. Imaging evaluation for acute pain in the right upper quadrant. *RadioGraphics*. 2004;24:1117–1135.

Bortoff GA, Chen MYM, Ott DJ, et al. Gallbladder stones: imaging and intervention. *RadioGraphics*. 2000;20:751–766.

# Case 150

## History

- 20-year-old man presenting with acute scrotal pain.

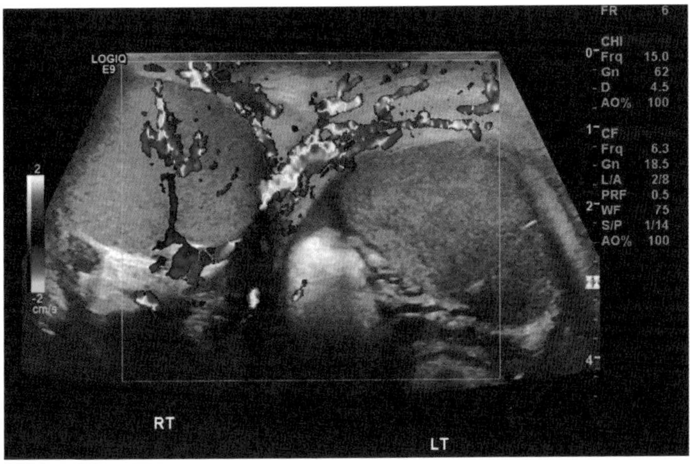


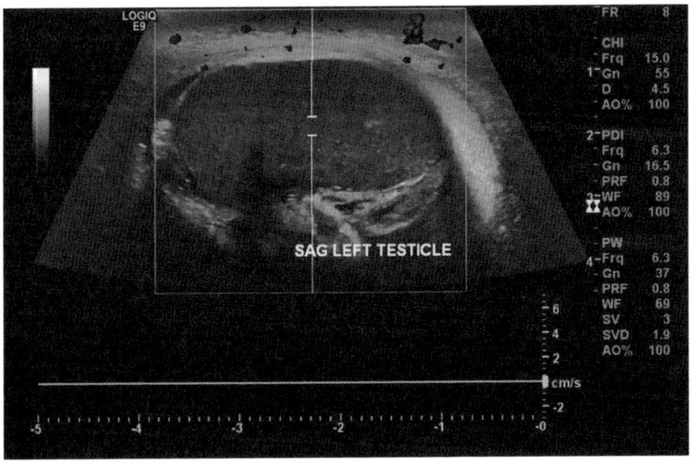


**Figures 150.1–150.2**

# Case 150  Testicular Torsion

## Findings

▶ Duplex ultrasonography is the main imaging modality used for the evaluation of acute scrotum.
▶ The most important finding is decreased or absent testicular blood flow and identification of the torsion knot in the spermatic cord located in the inguinoscrotal region above the testis and epididymis.
▶ The identification of a twisted cord with intratesticular blood flow is a sign that the testis is viable and may be salvaged after reduction and orchidopexy.
▶ Immediately after torsion (up to 3 h), testis volume and echogenicity may be normal.
▶ Later, an increase in testicular volume and hypoechogenicity or heterogeneous echogenicity, or both, may be detected.
▶ Cystic areas may be seen in the late phase.

## Differential Diagnosis

▶ Torsion of the appendix testis
▶ Epididymitis and epididymoorchitis
▶ Testicular trauma
▶ Idiopathic scrotal edema
▶ Inguinoscrotal hernia
▶ Testicular subtorsion
▶ Tunica vaginalis inflammation
▶ Abnormal processus vaginalis
▶ Hydrocele
▶ Varicocele/thrombosed varicocele
▶ Vasculitis (e.g., Schönlein-Henoch purpura)

## Presentation

▶ Acute scrotal pain ± nausea and vomiting
▶ Swollen/erythematous hemiscrotum/testicle
▶ Retracted testis
▶ Decreased or absent cremasteric reflex
▶ The testis is painful to palpation and may be transversely oriented inside the scrotal sac

## Management

▶ Surgical detorsion and orchiopexy of both testes
▶ Orchidectomy if the testes are necrotic and nonviable

## Teaching Points

▶ It has two peak incidences: a small one in the neonatal period and a large one during puberty, but it can occur at any age.
▶ This is a true surgical emergency, delay in its diagnosis may result in loss of a testis because of irreversible ischemia and the viability of a torsed testicle is dependent on the duration and completeness of torsion.
▶ Detorsion within 4–8 hours has generally been accepted as the optimal interval in which to salvage the affected testis.
▶ Surgery never should be delayed on the assumption of nonviability based on a clinical estimate of duration of torsion.
▶ If based on the history and examination the potential risk of testicular torsion remains, surgical exploration may be appropriate despite apparently normal imaging studies.

# Part III

# Pediatric

## History

▸ None

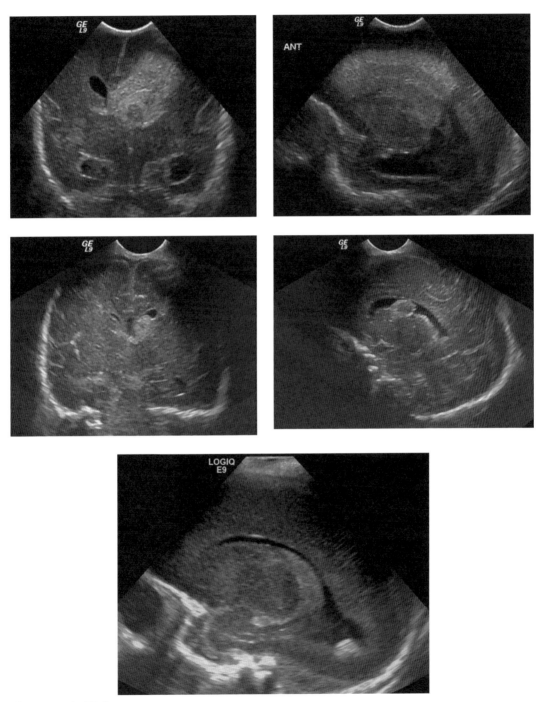

**Figures 151.1–151.5**

# Case 151  Germinal Matrix Hemorrhage

## Findings

### Cranial US

▶ Regions of increased echogenicity (signifying hemorrhage) in the region of the caudothalamic groove
  ▪ Located between the caudate head and the thalamus
  ▪ Best seen in coronal and sagittal planes
  ▪ Common pitfall: normal echogenic choroid plexus, which remains posterior to the caudothalamic groove
▶ ± uniform echogenic material in the lateral ventricles, most commonly layering in the occipital horns
▶ ± hydrocephalus
▶ ± ill-defined echogenicity in the periventricular white matter
  ▪ May represent intraparenchymal extension of hemorrhage or periventricular leukomalacia
▶ Can be unilateral or bilateral

## Differential Diagnosis

▶ Periventricular leukomalacia

## Teaching Points

▶ Grading of GMH
  ▪ Grade I: Hemorrhage involves the subependymal matrix only
  ▪ Grade II: Intraventricular extension without ventricular enlargement
  ▪ Grade III: Intraventricular extension with ventricular enlargement
  ▪ Grade IV: Periventricular intraparenchymal extension
▶ Presentation
  ▪ Typically preterm infants (<32 weeks gestation and <1,500 g)
    ▪ Overall prevalence of 10%–15% in preterm infants <35 weeks
  ▪ Most GMHs occur within the first 3 days of life
  ▪ Often asymptomatic
▶ Complications
  ▪ Hydrocephalus: communicating or obstructive
  ▪ Venous infarction in the periventricular parenchyma
    ▪ May result in periventricular cyst formation and rarely a large porencephalic cyst
▶ Prognosis
  ▪ Grade I, II, and III: typically have a good prognosis
  ▪ Grade IV: >25% mortality rate, long-term deficits in >50%

## Management

▶ Routine screening for GMH in infants <30 weeks or <1,250 g at birth. Typical screening regimen
  ▪ First screening examination at 4–5 days of age, or sooner if clinical concern
  ▪ Second screening head ultrasound at ~36 weeks or at time of discharge
▶ Imaging follow-up of positive ultrasounds is dictated by clinical circumstances.
▶ Treatment options
  ▪ Antenatal corticosteroids may reduce the risk of GMH
  ▪ Treatment typically limited to supportive care
  ▪ Hydrocephalus treated with shunting

## History

▸ None

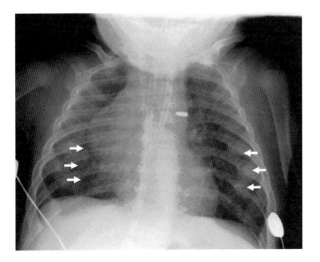

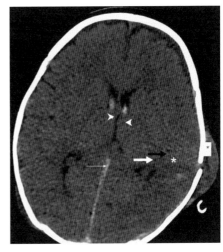

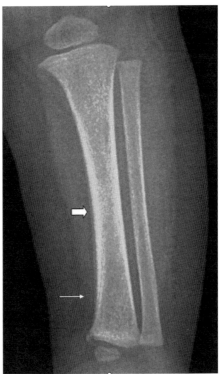

**Figures 152.1–152.3**

# Case 152   Nonaccidental Trauma, Child Abuse

## Findings

▶ Chest radiograph: Multiple rib fractures at various stages of healing (white arrows)
▶ Head CT: Subdural hemorrhage (thin white arrow), intraventricular hemorrhage (arrowheads), subarachnoid hemorrhage (thick white arrow), scalp hematoma (asterisk), skull fracture (black arrow)
▶ Tibia radiograph: Metaphyseal fracture/metaphyseal corner fracture/classic metaphyseal lesion (thin arrow), periosteal reaction (thick arrow)

## Differential Diagnosis

▶ Osteogenesis imprefecta
▶ Leukemia
▶ Spondylometaphyseal dysplasia

## Teaching Points

▶ Metaphyseal corner fractures are highly specific for nonaccidental trauma
▶ Other fractures highly specific for abuse include rib, sternum, scapula, and spinous processes

## Management

▶ Notify referring physician and/or child protection team about findings

### Further Readings

Kleinman PK; *Diagnostic Imaging of Child Abuse*. 2nd edition. St. Louis, MO: CV Mosby, Inc;1998.
Slovis TL, Coley BD, Bulas DI, Faerber FN. *Caffey's Pediatric Diagnostic Imaging*. 11th edn. Elsevier, Philadelphia, December, 2007.

## History

▸ 5-year-old boy with cough and fever.

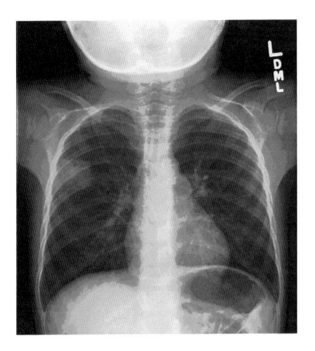

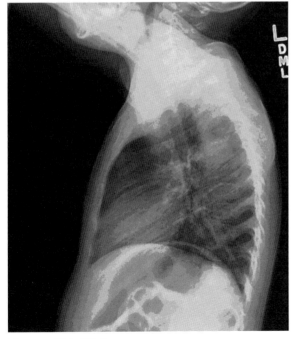

**Figures 153.1–153.2**

# Case 153   Round Pneumonia

## Findings

▶ Rounded opacity located in the superior segment of the right lower lobe

## Differential Diagnosis

▶ Metastatic disease
▶ Primary malignancy

## Teaching Points

▶ Common presentation of bacterial pneumonia in the pediatric population.
▶ Patient will present with common signs of pneumonia: cough, fever, and elevated WBC.

## Management

▶ Antibiotics
▶ Follow-up radiograph after treatment to ensure resolution

### Further Readings

Brant WE, Helms CA, eds. *Fundumentals of Diagnostic Radiology*. 3rd ed. Philadelphia: Lippincott Williams & Wilkins, 2006. p. 1252.
Pappas M, Yamato L, Anene O. *Pediatric radiology review*. New Jersey. Humana Press, 2007. p. 124.

## History

▶ 1.5-year-old boy with difficulty stridor.

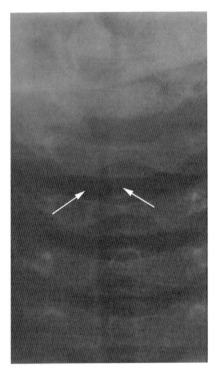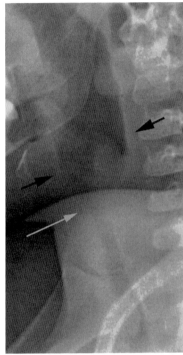

**Figures 154.1–154.2**

# Case 154  Croup

## Findings

### Frontal Radiograph

► "Steeple" or inverted "V" sign: Symmetric subglottic tracheal narrowing with loss of normal shouldering caused by subglottic edema

### Lateral Radiograph

► Inspiratory films: Hypopharyngeal distention (more common)
► Expiratory films: Hypopharyngeal collapse with overdistention of the lower cervical trachea
► Narrowing of the subglottic trachea with loss of definition
► Normal epiglottis and aryepiglottic folds.

## Differential Diagnosis

► Epiglottitis
► Foreign body aspiration
► Exudative tracheitis
► Subglottic hemangioma

## Teaching Points

► Radiography performed to exclude airway compromise from more serious causes of stridor
► Demographics
  ▪ 6 months–3 years (peak at 1 year)
  ▪ Typically younger than patients with epiglottitis (mean 3 years) or exudative tracheitis (6–10 years)
► Etiology
  ▪ Viral (parainfluenza virus most common)
► Epidemiology
  ▪ Most common cause of upper airway obstruction in young children
  ▪ Seasonal prevalence: Fall and Winter

## Management

► Usually benign, self-limited viral illness
► Oral or inhaled corticosteroids
► Inhaled epinephrine or intubation for severe cases

### Further Readings

Knutson D, Aring A. Viral croup. *Am Fam Physician*. 2004 Feb 1;69(3):535–40.
John SD, Swischuk LE: Stridor and upper airway obstruction in infants and children. *Radiographics*. 1992 Jul;12(4):625–43.

# Case 155

## History

▶ 18-year-old male presenting with high fever, sore throat, stridor, and drooling.

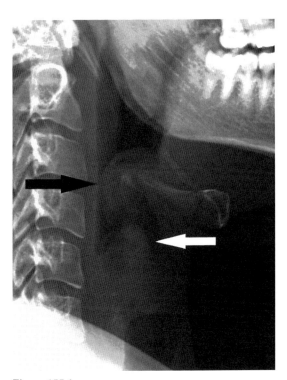

**Figure 155.1**

# Case 155  Epiglottitis

## Findings

▶ "Thumb sign": Marked enlargement of epiglottis on lateral radiograph (white arrow)
▶ Marked thickening and upward convexity of aryepiglottic folds (black arrow)
▶ May demonstrate hypopharyngeal widening and subglottic narrowing on AP view
▶ CT: Typically not necessary, but can assist with differential diagnosis and evaluation for emphysematous epiglottitis or an associated abscess
  ▪ Edematous low-attenuation swelling of the epiglottis and aryepiglottic folds, occasionally with an associated phlegmon

## Differential Diagnosis

▶ "Omega" epiglottis: Normal epiglottis imaged obliquely
▶ Croup
▶ Retropharyngeal abscess
▶ Exudative tracheitis

## Teaching Points

▶ Typically a lateral radiograph is the only imaging needed for diagnosis; the patient should be maintained in upright comfortable position for imaging
▶ Onset of total airway occlusion can be sudden, and is associated with agitation of the patient or airway; children are especially at risk
▶ Classically associated with *Haemophilus influenza* type b (Hib), but this etiology is much less common after introduction of Hib vaccine in 1985; now more likely to present from a wide range of pathogens
▶ Classically occurs in young children, but introduction of the Hib vaccine has resulted in a relative increase in adult presentation

## Management

▶ Steroids and wide-spectrum antibiotics
▶ Do not agitate the patient or airway, because this may precipitate sudden airway occlusion
▶ May require emergent intubation, ideally performed quickly by an experienced clinician

Further Readings

Capps EF, Kinsella JJ, Gupta M, et al. Emergency imaging assessment of acute, nontraumatic conditions of the head and neck. *RadioGraphics*. 2010;30(5):1335–1352.
Shah RK, Roberson DW, Jones DT. Epiglottitis in the *Hemophilus influenzae* type B vaccine era: changing trends. *Laryngoscope*. 2004;114(3):557–560.

## History

▶ 4-year-old boy with intermittent fever, nausea, vomiting, and neck pain.

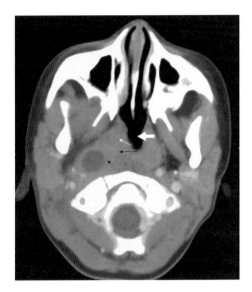 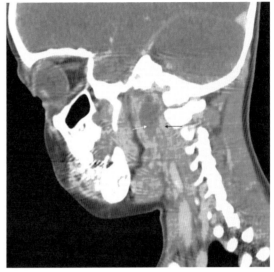

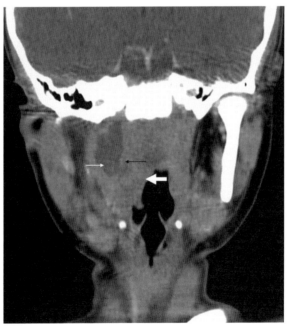

**Figures 156.1–156.3**

# Case 156 Retropharyngeal Abscess

## Findings

**CT**

▶ Low-attenuation collection in retropharyngeal/parapharyngeal soft tissues (black arrows)
▶ Peripheral enhancing wall
▶ May contain gas
▶ Effacement of fat planes
▶ Mass effect on adjacent airway
▶ May compress or invade regional vasculature, thrombophlebitis (Lemierre syndrome)

**Radiograph**

▶ Enlarged prevertebral, retropharyngeal soft tissues
▶ May contain gas
▶ Mass effect on airway
▶ May be normal

## Differential Diagnosis

▶ Pseudothickening of the prevertebral soft tissues related to short necks in infants expiratory phase or neck flexion

## Teaching Points

▶ Prevertebral soft tissue should not be greater than AP diameter of vertebral bodies
▶ Anterior border of soft tissues may be convex
▶ Gas in soft tissues indicates abscess, but often no gas is seen and radiographs cannot differentiate between an abscess and phlegmon

## Management

▶ Antibiotics, surgical drainage, aspiration, maintain airway

Further Reading

Slovis TL, Coley BD, Bulas DI, Faerber EN. *Caffey's Pediatric Diagnostic Imaging*. 11th edn. Elsevier, Philadelphia, December, 2007.

## History

▸ Cough wheezing

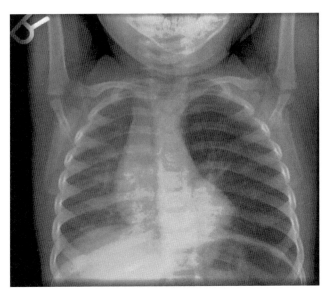

**Figure 157.1**

# Case 157  Bronchial Foreign Body

## Findings

### Chest Radiograph

- Asymmetric lung volumes (left greater than right)
- Hyperlucency (left lung)
- Oligemia (left lung)
- Mediastinal shift
- Static lung volumes on inspiration/expiration and decubitus images

## Differential Diagnosis

- Viral pneumonia, asthma, endobronchial mass

## Teaching Points

- Often difficult to obtain inspiration and expiration views because of young age and inability to cooperate. In these cases obtain lateral decubitus views
- Lateral decubitus view, the dependent lung should collapse, consider chest fluoroscopy
- Most foreign bodies are organic (peanut most common) and are not radiopaque
- Chest radiographs may be normal, show air trapping, atelectasis, and mediastinal shift

## Management

- Foreign body removal

## Further Reading

Donnelly LF, Jones BV, O'Hara SM, et al. *Diagnostic imaging : Pediatrics* (2nd Ed.) Springer; Amysis, Salt Lake City (Utah) 2011
Slovis TL, Coley BD, Bulas DI, Faerber EN. *Caffey's Pediatric Diagnostic Imaging.* 11th edn. Elsevier, Philadelphia,December, 2007.

## History

► 10 day old, born at 30 weeks gestation, feeding intolerance

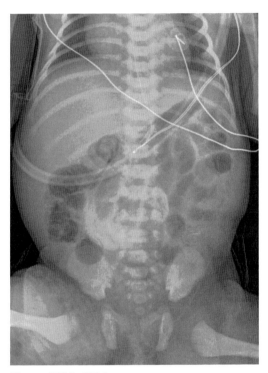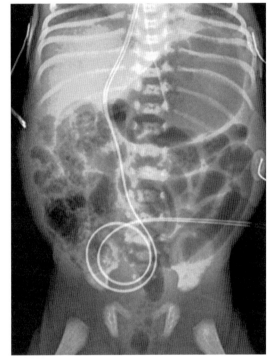

**Figures 158.1–158.2**

# Case 158  Necrotizing Enterocolitis

## Findings

- ▶ Pneumatosis intestinalis
- ▶ Distended loops of bowel
- ▶ Portal venous gas
- ▶ Differential diagnosis
- ▶ Ileus

## Teaching Points

- ▶ Pneumatosis may be linear or bubbly and is diagnostic of NEC
- ▶ First sign is often dilated loop or loops of bowel, most common in right lower quadrant, loops may be stacked
- ▶ Fixed loop of dilated bowel not changing over time is worrisome for NEC
- ▶ If pneumoperitoneum is suspected, do left later decubitus to better detect free air adjacent to liver

## Management

- ▶ Serial KUBs for follow-up, NPO, surgical consultation

Further Readings

Donnelly LF, Jones BV, O'Hara SM, et al. *Diagnostic imaging : Pediatrics* (2nd Ed.) Springer; Amysis, Salt Lake City (Utah) 2011.

Slovis TL, Coley BD, Bulas DI, Faerber EN. *Caffey's Pediatric Diagnostic Imaging.* 11th edn. Elsevier, Philadelphia,December, 2007.

## History

▶ Bilious vomiting.

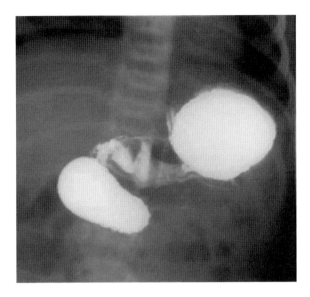 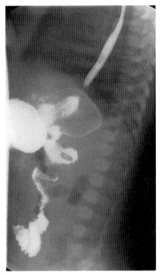

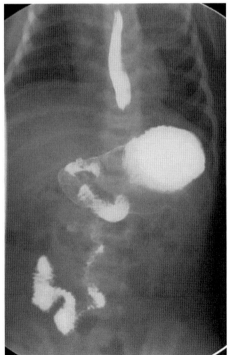

**Figures 159.1–159.3**

# Case 159  Malrotation and Midgut Volvulus

### Findings

- Abnormal position of the duodenal-jejunal junction
- Spiraling of descending duodenum is diagnostic of volvulus
- Distended duodenal bulb, distended proximal duodenum Differential Diagnosis
- Pseudomalrotation, duodenal-jejunal junction (DJJ) displaced may be gastric or bowel distention, if suspected repeat UGI when contrast has cleared
- If spiraling not seen, duodenal atresia or duodenal web

### Teaching Points

- Malrotation is diagnosed on an upper GI when the DJJ does not meet the normal criteria
- Normal DJJ is to the left of the spine at the level of the duodenal bulb

### Management

- Notify referring physician and/or pediatric surgery about findings.
- If malrotation is present this is a true surgical emergency

### Further Readings

Swischuk LE (Ed.), *Imaging of the Newborn, Infant and Young Child* (4th edn), William and Wilkins, Baltimore, MD (1997).
Kleinman PK; *Diagnostic Imaging of Child Abuse.* 2nd edition. St. Louis, MO: CV Mosby, Inc;1998.
Slovis TL, Coley BD, Bulas DI, Faerber EN. *Caffey's Pediatric Diagnostic Imaging.* 11th edn. Elsevier, Philadelphia, December, 2007.

## History

▶ 10-month-old boy with abdominal pain and vomiting.

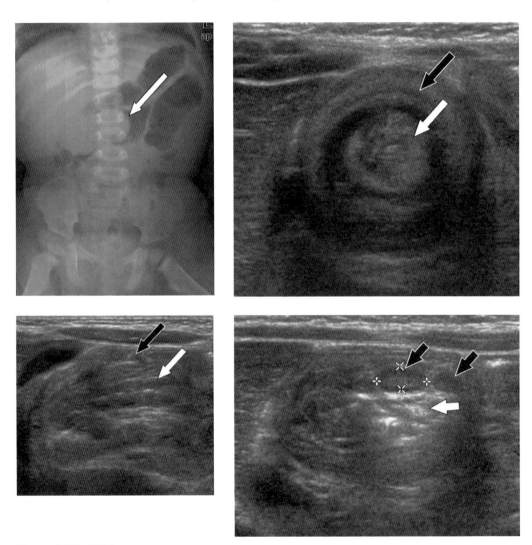

**Figures 160.1–160.4**

# Case 160  Intussusception

## Findings

- ▶ Abdominal radiograph: rounded filling defect, soft tissue mass (white arrow) within the colonic gas, nonvisualization of air-filled cecum on right side up lateral decubitus radiograph
- ▶ Sonography: bowel within bowel or target sign, concentric layers representing bowel (intussusceptum; white arrows) surrounded by bowel (intussuscipiens; black arrows), pseudokidney appearance on longitudinal images, fat (short white arrow) and lymph nodes (short black arrows) between the two bowel loops

## Differential Diagnosis

- ▶ Appendicitis
- ▶ Gastroenteritis
- ▶ Meckel diverticulum
- ▶ Ovarian pathology

## Teaching Points

- ▶ Defined by the invagination of a part of the intestine into itself where a proximal segment of bowel (the intussusceptum) telescopes into a distal segment (the intussuscipiens), dragging associated mesentery with it
- ▶ Consequent development of venous and lymphatic congestion results in intestinal edema, which can ultimately lead to ischemia, perforation, and peritonitis
- ▶ Occurs most often near the ileocecal junction without an identifiable lead point
- ▶ A common cause of acute abdomen, particularly in children younger than 2 years of age

## Management

- ▶ Retrograde pressure can be exerted using air or water-soluble medium in an enema reduction to reduce the intussusception
- ▶ Surgical intervention may be required if symptoms are protracted, there are signs of peritonitis, or enema reduction is unsuccessful

### Further Readings

Byrne AT, Geoghegan T, Govender P, et al. The imaging of intussusception. *Clin Radiol.* 2005;60:39–46.
Daneman A, Navarro O. Intussusception Part 1: review of diagnostic approaches. *Pediatr Radiol.* 2003;33:79–85.

## History

▸ 12-year-old female with traumatic ankle pain and swelling.

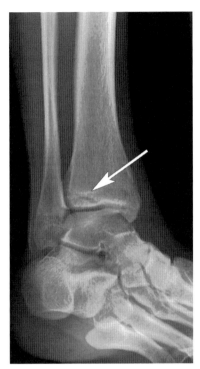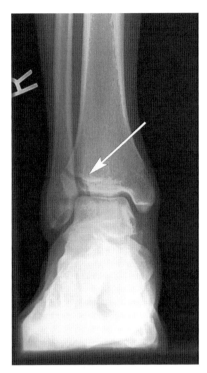

**Figures 161.1–161.2**

# Case 161  Salter-Harris Fracture Type III (Juvenile Tillaux Fracture)

## Findings

### Radiographs

▶ Type I: Occult or physeal widening
▶ Type II: Fracture extending from the metaphysis to the physis
▶ Type III: Fracture extending from the epiphysis to the physis
▶ Type IV: Fracture extending through the epiphysis, physis, and metaphysis
▶ Type V: Narrowing of the physis

### CT

▶ Used to evaluate extent of fracture and degree of displacement

### MRI

▶ Increased T2 signal at physis
▶ Hypointense fracture line on T1 and T2 weight sequences with surrounding bone marrow edema

## Differential Diagnosis

▶ Ankle sprain
▶ Stress injury
▶ Triplane fracture

## Teaching Points

▶ Type I fractures may be radiographically occult or show physeal widening
   ▪ Consider comparison with contralateral limb
▶ Type II fracture most common (>70%)
   ▪ Except distal humerus where most are type IV
   ▪ Good prognosis
▶ Type III and Type IV more prone to chronic disability
▶ Type V associated with growth disturbances
▶ Complications
   ▪ Premature epiphyseal closure with limb shortening
   ▪ Joint incongruity
   ▪ Trapped periosteum
   ▪ More common with knee and ankle fractures
▶ Juvenile tillaux fracture (current case)
   ▪ Exclusive type of fracture occurring in adolescence before complete fusion of the tibial growth plate
   ▪ The tibial growth plate fuses from medial to lateral
   ▪ Common age of incidence is 11–15 years (male mean age of 14 years; female mean age of 12 years)

## Management

▶ Casting for low-grade Salter-Harris categories
▶ Open reduction and internal fixation for high-grade Salter-Harris categories

## Further Readings

Barmada A, Gaynor T, Mubarak SJ, et al. Premature physeal closure following distal tibia physeal fractures: a new radiographic predictor. *J Pediatr Orthop*. 2003 Nov-Dec;23(6):733–739.
Resnik CS. Diagnostic imaging of pediatric skeletal trauma. *Radiol Clin North Am*. 1989 Sep;27(5):1013–1022.

## History

▸ None

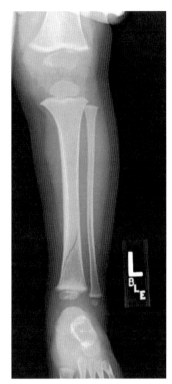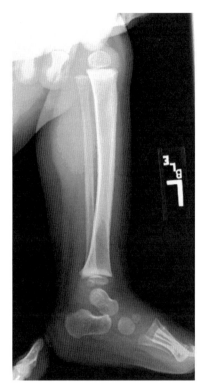

**Figures 162.1–162.2**

# Case 162   Toddler's Fracture

## Findings

▶ Spiral nondisplaced fracture of the mid tibial shaft

## Differential Diagnosis

▶ Nonaccidental trauma (typically midshaft or upper one-third of tibia), whereas toddler fractures are typically midshaft or lower one-third of tibia

▶ Osteomyelitis (in cases where fracture is occult and there are clinical signs of infection)

## Teaching Points

▶ Etiology: Typically a toddler (1–2 years old, usually under 3 years old) undergoes a rotational twisting force as he or she stumbles, falls, or gets foot stuck against an object

▶ Presentation: Refusal to bear weight or walk

▶ Clinical examination: Gently twisting foot with knee in fixed position elicits pain

▶ Further studies: Need two views—the fracture may only be seen on one view; internal oblique view may be the most sensitive. Tc MDP scan is sensitive but nonspecific and exposes to additional radiation

▶ Other
  ▪ Can occur in the calcaneus and cuboid
  ▪ Frequently occult (up to 43% of time), so low threshold for long leg cast

## Management

▶ Long leg cast for 2–3 weeks

### Further Readings

Halsey MF, Finzel KC, Carrion WV, et al. Toddler's fracture: presumptive diagnosis and treatment. *J Pediatr Orthop.* 2001;21:152–156.

Lonergan GJ, Baker AM, Morey MK, et al. From the Archives of the AFIP: Child abuse: radiologic-pathologic correlation. *RadioGraphics.* 2003;23:811–845.

## History

▸ 10-year-old girl status post fall.

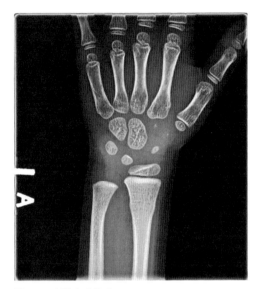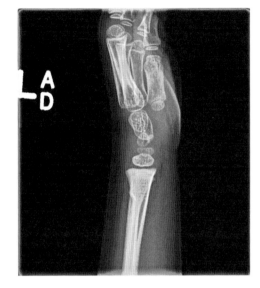

**Figures 163.1–163.2**

# Case 163   Torus/Buckle Fractures

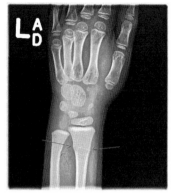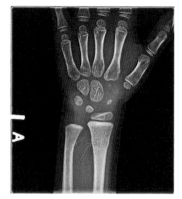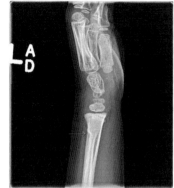

**Figures 163.3–163.5**

## Findings

▶ Oblique view demonstrating cortical irregularity of the distal radius and ulna (Figure 163.1)
▶ Lateral view demonstrating cortical irregularity of the distal radius and ulna with volar angulation of the distal radius fracture (Figure 163.2)
▶ Oblique view with white arrows denoting fracture sites (Figure 163.3)
▶ AP view with white arrows demonstrating cortical irregularity of the distal radius and ulna (Figure 163.4)
▶ Lateral view with open black arrow demonstrating "dinner fork deformity" (Figure 163.4)

## Differential diagnosis

None

## Teaching Points

▶ Most common location is in the distal radius
▶ Usually caused by fall on outstretched hand
▶ More common with low-energy injuries compared with displaced fractures, which usually result from higher energy mechanisms
▶ Caused by highly cellular and porous pediatric bone with a large amount of collagen and cartilage, and thicker and stronger periosteum compared with adults
▶ Patient may have a "dinner fork" deformity seen on lateral view (see Figure 163.4)

## Management

▶ Buckle fractures are usually treated with short arm casts

## Further Reading

Carson S, Woolridge D, Colleti J, Kilgore K. Pediatric upper extremity injuries. *Pediatr Clin North Am.* 2006 Feb;53(1):41–67, v.

## History

► 4-year-old boy with wheeze.

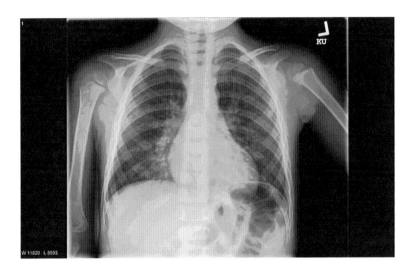

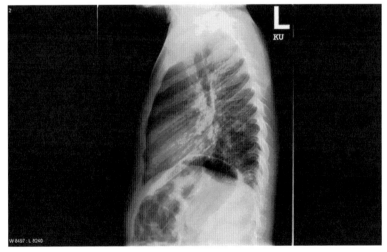

**Figures 164.1–164.2**

# Case 164   Viral pneumonia

**Findings**

▸ PA and lateral chest radiographs, respectively, demonstrate bilateral hilar opacities

**Differential Diagnosis**

▸ Viral pneumonia
▸ Reactive airway disease
▸ Bacterial pneumonia

**Teaching Points**

▸ Viruses are common pathogen in pediatric population, especially the first 2 years of life, including RSV, influenza, and adenovirus
▸ Radiographic findings: bilateral hilar opacities, peribronchiole cuffing, atelectasis and/or hyperinflation

**Management**

▸ Outpatient therapy is adequate if the child does not have respiratory or feeding difficulties
▸ Bronchodilators may be used especially with bronchiolitis-like symptoms

Further Reading

Pappas, Michael, Yamato, Loren, Anene, Okechukwu. *Pediatric radiology review*. New Jersey. Humana Press, 2007. p. 123.

# Index of Cases

# Index

Hematuria, 105–106
Hemopericardium, 81–82
Hemoperitoneum, 111–112
Hemorrhage
    adrenal, 102
    aneurysm, 201–202
    germinal matrix, 327–328
    intracerebral, 203–204
    subarachnoid, 11–12, 202
    thalamic, 204
    ventricular, 204
Hemothorax, 69–70
Hepatitis, 271–272
Herniation, intracranial, 17–18
Hindfoot trauma, 173–174
Hip dislocation, 183–184
HIV infection, 197–198
Humerus fractures, proximal, 133–134
Humpback deformity, 144
Hydrosalpinx, 319–320
Hyperflexion injury
    of cervical spine, 53, 54
    of spine, 53–54
Hypertensive intracerebral hemorrhage,
    203–204
Hypotension, intracranial, 213–214
Hypoxic ischemic injury, 215–216

IJVT (internal jugular venous thrombosis),
    221–222
Ileus, adynamic, 300
Iliac fractures, 158
Incudomalleolar joint subluxation or
    dislocation, 24
Incudostapedial joint separation, 24
Incus dislocation, 24
Infarctions, spinal cord, 239–240
Inflammatory bowel disease, 299–300
Inhalation
    smoke, 265–266
    toxic, 265–266
Internal carotid artery dissection, 60
Internal jugular venous thrombosis (IJVT),
    221–222
Intertrochanteric fracture, 163–164
Intoxication, ethanol, 19
Intracerebral hemorrhage, hypertensive,
    203–204
Intracranial aneurysm, 202
Intracranial herniation, 17–18
Intracranial hypotension, 213–214

Intramural hematoma, aortic, 261–262
Intraperitoneal bladder rupture, 104,
    105–106
Intratesticular hematoma, 110
Intussusception, 291–292
    pediatric, 345–346
Ischemic colitis, 295–296
Ischemic injury, hypoxic, 215–216

Jefferson fracture, 41–42
Jones fracture, 176
Juvenile tillaux fracture (Salter-Harris
    fracture Type III), 347–348

Kidney. *see under* Renal
Kidney stones, 309–310
Knee dislocation, posterior, 167–168
Knee pain, 179–180
Knee trauma, 165–166

Laceration
    liver, 90
    lung, 73–74
    renal, 119–120
    splenic, 117–118
Lateral compression fracture, 157–158
Lateral malleolus fracture, 186
Lauge-Hansen classification, 186
Le Fort maxillary fracture, 35–36
    Le Fort I, 36
    Le Fort II, 35, 36
    Le Fort III, 36
Left flank pain, 309–310
Left knee trauma, 165–166
Left lower quadrant pain, 289–290
Left-sided chest pain, 73–74
Left-sided nasal orbital ethmoid
    fracture, 29–30
Left vertebral artery dissection, 59, 60
Leg pain, 255–256
Lemierre syndrome, 222
Letournel's classification system, 160
Leukemia, acute myelocytic, 301–302
Lipohemarthrosis, 170
Lisfranc injury, 177–178
Lisfranc (tarsometatarsal) joint fracture
    dislocation, 178
Liver abscess, 315–316
Liver injury, traumatic, 89–90
Lobar collapse, 263–264
Lobar pneumonia, 251, 252